# Including me

*Managing complex health needs
in schools and early years settings*

**Council for
Disabled
Children**

department for
**education and skills**

This book was written in partnership with

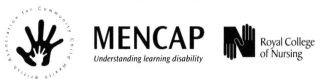

ISBN 1-904787-60-6
© The Council for Disabled Children 2005
Designed by Susan Clarke for Expression, IP23 8HH

### Disclaimer

This handbook is intended as guidance only and should not be treated as an authoritative interpretation of the law, which is a matter for the courts.

The forms, protocols and other documents included in the handbook are developed by local authorities, trusts and other providers and are intended to illustrate the main text. The content does not necessarily reflect the views of the DfES or Council for Disabled Children.

### Photocopying

The forms in this book can be photocopied and adapted for local services and settings.

### About the Council for Disabled Children (CDC)

The Council for Disabled Children provides a national forum for the discussion and development of a wide range of policy and practice issues relating to service provision and support for disabled children and young people and those with special educational needs.

Our membership is drawn from a wide range of professional, voluntary and statutory organisations, including parent representatives and representatives of disabled people. This ensures we have a good balance of interests and expertise.

Our broad based membership and extensive network of contacts gives us a unique overview of current issues. It also helps us promote collaborative and partnership working among organisations, and develop quality support for disabled children and their families.

For more information on CDC please see our website at www.ncb.org.uk/cdc

Council for Disabled Children
National Children's Bureau
8 Wakley Street
London
EC1V 7QE
020 7843 6334

# Including me

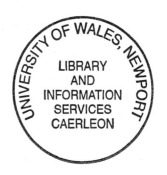

# Contents

# Acknowledgements

This handbook was written by Jeanne Carlin, Freelance Disability Consultant. The handbook brings together information and good practice from a number of areas across the country. The writing of this handbook would therefore not have been possible without the help and support of a large number of individuals and organisations.

Acknowledgement and thanks needs to go to the following:
- Members of the advisory group – Christine Lenehan (Council for Disabled Children), Beverley Dawkins (Mencap), Mark Whiting (RCN), Gail Treml and Phil Snell (DfES), David Vickers (BACCH) and Ian Southern (Lancashire Local Authority).
- Members of the Health Needs in Education consortium for their support and advice.
- The Department for Education and Skills for funding the work.
- Mark Whiting, Gaynor Evans, Janette Harrison, Lucy Wills, Karen Woollard (Hertfordshire Partnership NHS Trust) and Wendy Faulknall (Queen Elizabeth Hospital, London) for writing the five exemplars.
- Philippa Stobbs (Council for Disabled Children) for writing the information relating to the Disability Discrimination Act.

In addition, our thanks to the local authorities, health trusts and other organisations and individuals who sent us examples of protocols and good practice and invited the author to visit them in order to develop the information which is produced in the handbook. The fact that all the material is not reproduced here is not an indication of quality but of our need to select information which illustrated the text and represented the process. We have identified the source of all the material used in the handbook.

A particular thanks go to Sally and her parents for their kind permission to reproduce Sally's story and the delightful cover photo.

Finally, our thanks to all the children and their parents who gave consent for their information to be used in the case studies or provided the inspiration for the writing of this material.

We hope this handbook provides the practical information which will assist you to ensure that children with complex health needs are included in schools and early years settings.

# Foreword

Lord Andrew Adonis

The Green Paper *Every Child Matters* signalled the Government's commitment to helping every child to:
- be healthy
- stay safe
- enjoy and achieve
- make a positive contribution, and
- achieve economic well being.

150 local change programmes, one in every local authority area, are working to turn this commitment into a reality, bringing services for children and families together and making them more accessible.

The Children's National Service Framework sets national outcome standards for health and social services and their interface with education and *Removing Barriers to Achievement*, our special educational needs (SEN) strategy, sets out a long-term programme of action to improve outcomes for children with SEN and disabilities, some of whom will have complex health needs.

We know that children with complex health needs can miss out on opportunities other children take for granted because they do not always get the support they need. It is essential that local authorities and schools have policies and protocols in place to ensure that the needs of these children are addressed, so that they can take part in activities with their peers.

*Including me* contains practical examples illustrating how local authorities have developed effective policies for supporting children with complex health needs in maintaining their health and accessing the curriculum. It also contains case studies to show how the positive difference this makes to the lives of these children and young people. The information in *Including me* will help local authorities, schools and early years settings to review their practice and develop their policies.

I commend it to you as a welcome source of useful ideas.

*Parliamentary Under Secretary of State for Schools*

# Introduction

## Who is this handbook for?

**Including me** will help local authorities, schools, early years settings, and health providers develop policies and procedures specific to local circumstances, so that children and young people with complex health needs can access education and childcare. It draws on examples of good practice from across the country. These examples illustrate the ways in which health, education and other setting staff can work together to develop local policies and procedures to ensure that the needs of this group of children are met in a co-ordinated and child-centred way.

## To which children does this guidance relate?

**Including me** is concerned with children and young people from birth to 19 years of age who have complex health needs and as a consequence require additional support and/or care within the school or early years setting in order to:
- maintain optimal health during the day
- access the curriculum to the maximum extent

Many children within this group will be 'technology dependent', that is, they will depend on a technological device to sustain life or optimise health, *and* need regular and complex care for substantial parts of the day and night.

Examples of care or health needs for which children might require additional support include:
- Restricted mobility
  *for example a child with physical impairments who uses a wheelchair*
- Difficulty in breathing
  *for example a child with a tracheostomy who requires regular airway suctioning during the day*
- Problems with eating and drinking
  *for example a child who requires a gastrostomy feed at lunch time*
- Continence problems
  *for example a child who requires assistance with bladder emptying and needs catheterisation at each break time*
- Susceptibility to infection
  *for example a child who is receiving steroid therapy*

This list is provided for illustrative purposes only and **is not comprehensive.**

Detailed case studies based upon these illustrative examples are provided in the exemplars in Appendix 1.

Not all children with complex health care needs will be disabled, nor will they all have special educational needs. The diagram below represents the overlap between these three groups of children:

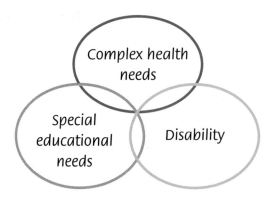

Disabled children with complex health care needs will have additional rights under the disability legislation, which is outlined in Appendix 2. Information on prevalence of complex health needs from national research is detailed in Appendix 3.

## Which settings?

This handbook has been written for the following settings:
- all schools
  - maintained, non-maintained and independent
  - mainstream and special
  - day and residential
- early years settings (provided by the local authority, private or voluntary organisations), including
  - children's centres
  - Sure Start local programmes
  - childminders
  - play groups
  - nursery schools
- other settings (provided by the local authority, private or voluntary organisations), including
  - before- and after-school clubs
  - holiday play schemes

## How to use this handbook

**Including me** follows the process of developing policies, protocols and practice for supporting children with complex health needs.

Each step in the process is a short chapter, which may contain additional forms, protocols or examples to illustrate that stage of the process. Five exemplars (in Appendix 1) based on real-life case examples illustrate the factors and issues which may need to be considered at each stage in this process.

- *developing local authority policies through partnerships*
- *schools and early years perspectives*
- *anticipatory duties, planning and reasonable adjustments*
- *admissions*
- *risk management and assessments*
- *health care plans*
- *training of staff*
- *support arrangements*

# 1  Developing local authority policies through partnerships

« Local health agencies, local authorities and schools work closely to ensure that children with complex medical regimes, whether through chronic ill health or disability, receive the specific support they need so that they can attend school – whether a special school or mainstream – on a regular basis. Where support is provided by school staff, they are fully trained by health professionals. »

(National Service Framework for Children, Young People and Maternity Services, DfES/DH, 2004, p.24)

How can local authorities and other employers, responsible for schools, early years and other settings ensure that the support described in the National Service Framework (NSF) is available?

Across the country a number of local authorities have developed partnership arrangements with their local health providers and written joint policies and protocols. All employers, both local authorities and others should develop policies which are in line with statutory responsibilities and reflect local needs and resources. The guidance, *Managing Medicines in Schools and Early Years Settings* (DfES/DH, 2005) outlines the roles and responsibilities of local authorities and other employers, schools and governing bodies, early years settings and management groups, staff and parents. The same responsibilities will apply to managing complex health needs.

Policies and protocols should take into account any standard or inspection framework which applies to that particular school or setting. These policies and protocols should reflect good practice, develop opportunities for inclusion and be child-centred in their approach.

### What needs to take place?

Policies and protocols should:
- be developed through joint working between education and health. Other sections of Children's Service departments, for example social services as well as the voluntary sector may be included. This work may be developed through meetings, focus groups, consultation workshops and small working parties
- involve local authority staff, head teachers, SENCOs, early years staff, health and safety officers, SEN advisors, children's community

nurses, school nurses, doctors, community paediatricians, staff from health trusts and relevant local teacher associations or unions from an early stage rather than consulting them at the end of the process
- be rolled out to schools and early years settings and shared with governing bodies and management groups
- be monitored by a multi-agency group involving the major stakeholders
- be updated based on the experience of schools and early years settings and as technology and medical information develops

## Why is a joint approach necessary?

A joint approach:
- promotes consistency of approach across a local authority area and gives status to that approach
- ensures the commitment of all agencies to providing shared governance and shared ownership of the process
- draws on the expertise and knowledge of staff in all agencies
- ensures that the roles and responsibilities of all agencies are clearly defined
- lessens confusion for parents about what tasks schools and early years settings can and cannot take on
- helps to clarify the entitlement to a level of support a child with complex health needs may expect

Joint arrangements for supporting children should cover funding.

The local authority has a responsibility to ensure that early years settings get advice on managing medicines and complex health needs.

In some areas this type of partnership working has taken place between the education authority and health providers and in other areas the partnership has been across all agencies: education, health, social services and the voluntary sector. Two examples of this type of joint approach are provided below.

**example** *Lancashire local education authority* *established a medical support working group, bringing together various LEA officers and advisors, a couple of headteachers, teacher associations and other union representatives and colleagues from local area health authorities (as they were known at the time), including a community paediatrician, school nursing manager and specialist health visitor. The main task of the group was to create a document of advice and guidance for headteachers on the administration of medication in schools and on supporting pupils who have health needs. Over a period of two years the working group split into a number of sub-groups to prepare and write the document, with an officer from the LEA acting as editor to collate all the contributions into an unified whole. A copy of the completed document or guide together* with an accompanying video was sent to every maintained school and each school nursing team in the county. The video explains succinctly the legislation and guidance as well as the roles and responsibilities of the LEA, the school and its staff in relation to children with health needs. The guide provides more practical information and forms which can be used and adapted by schools as well as information on various medical conditions.

The experience of the group was that it was essential for education and health to work together on this guide, with each party contributing their own perspective and expertise. The teacher union representatives on the working group played a crucial role in allaying the fears of their colleagues within the unions and helped to define shared responsibilities for these issues. When the materials were published they had the support of all the teacher unions.

The medical support working group continues to meet on an 'as necessary' basis to review general issues concerning support for pupils who have health needs and to provide additional guidance materials to schools. The additional guidance produced by the group has included subject areas such as chronic fatigue syndrome, HIV/AIDS, toileting and continence and MRSA.

**example** In **Bath and North East Somerset**, a small working group was set up to develop policy and guidelines for staff working with children who require invasive procedures to meet their individual medical needs. This group of children need support that routinely crosses agencies and professional boundaries, therefore the working group consisted of representatives from the local authority education health and safety team and social services and the NHS school nurses and lifetime nurses. The objective was to ensure that the procedures and the high quality of support were the same for all children served by the local authority and the primary care trust, no matter which setting or who was the carer. These ranged from nurseries and schools to parents and foster carers.

The group met for about 18 months and each representative was able to contribute their unique knowledge and experience to the development of a document. This was vital, to prevent inaccurate assumptions being made about the settings or staff with which the other contributors worked. The completed document contained amongst other things, the legal background, key principles such as the social model of disability, and defined those techniques which may be carried out by trained lay carers and those which should only be carried out by medical personnel. This was supplemented with the appropriate care plans and training competence and parental permission forms.

Guidance of course, is not enough. It must be supported by training and agreement between members of the working group on training was drawn up. Training on medical techniques for all carers is carried out by the NHS staff, but the local authority staff are able to contribute training on 'safer people handling' where this is required.

Widespread consultation on the completed policy and guidelines amongst interested groups, including the trade unions, resulted in some refinement to clarify the details. After which the policy and guidance on invasive medical procedures were finally distributed and were very well received. The LEA has subsequently consulted health service partners on their revised 'Guidance to schools on the administration of medication', which covered the handling of routine requests to administer medication in schools, as opposed to the use of invasive procedures for children with a chronic medical condition.

Arrangements were put in place to ensure that the local authority was notified each year of new entrants to mainstream school or children with complex health needs who were transferring from infants to junior schools or from primary to secondary schools. These arrangements are detailed in chapter 3.

# 2 Schools and early years perspectives

> « All of our pupils have some level of physical disability but many have associated learning, sensory or other medical related difficulties. This means we need to have a range of procedures in place to ensure pupils' individual needs are identified and met to guarantee maximum access to the curriculum and learning opportunities. »
>
> Victoria School (special school in Birmingham)

> « This school promotes inclusion and will take all reasonable steps to ensure that children/young people with a disability or SEN are not discriminated against or treated less favourably than other pupils. The school will work in partnership with the family and other agencies in the best interests of the pupil and to maximise educational opportunity. »
>
> The Learning Trust, Hackney, draft sample statement for schools

Each school, early years and other setting should have in place a policy and protocols on supporting children with complex health needs. The policy must be in line with the policy of the employer, most frequently the local authority; this also ensures consistency and clarity across all settings. It could be a stand alone document but it need not be; it could, for example be part of an overall Health and Safety Policy, inclusion policy or medical needs policy.

### Why should schools and early years settings have a policy in relation to complex health needs?

A policy will:
- demonstrate the commitment to positively promoting the inclusion of children with complex health needs
- lead to a clear understanding of the roles and responsibilities of staff within a school or early years setting
- clarify for parents and children what they can expect from the school or early years settings and what is expected from them

### What should a policy contain?

A policy should contain information on:

- the roles and responsibilities of staff with regard to supporting children with complex health needs
- what the school or early years setting expects from the parents in terms of being kept informed and updated about their child's health needs
- the training which staff can expect to receive prior to supporting a child with complex health needs
- indemnity or insurance arrangements
- risk management, record keeping and protocols to be followed
- responses to emergency situations
- any additional arrangements which need to be in place for activities which take place away from the usual school or other setting site

### Which issues should be clarified?[1]

### Roles and responsibilities

The role of staff in administering medicines in schools and early years settings, is as follows:

> Teachers' conditions of employment do not include giving or supervising a pupil taking medicines. The only exceptions are set out in the paragraph below. Schools should ensure that they have sufficient members of support staff who are employed and appropriately trained to manage medicines as part of their duties.

> For registered day care the conditions of employment are individual to each setting. It is therefore for the registered person to arrange who should administer medicines within a setting, either on a voluntary basis or as part of a contract of employment.

Similar issues are involved in managing complex health needs. Most settings employ support staff with job descriptions written to cover the tasks required to support this group of children.

### Duty of care

Duty of care is explained as follows:

> Anyone caring for children, including teachers, other school staff and day care staff have a common law duty of care to act like any reasonable prudent parent. Staff need to make sure that children are healthy and safe. In exceptional circumstance the duty of care could extend to administering medicines and/or taking action in an emergency. This duty extends to staff leading activities taking place off site such as visits, outings or field trips.

### Indemnity

> With the exception of local authorities, employers must take out employer's liability insurance to provide cover for injury to staff acting

1 Quotations are from: Department for Education and Skills and Department of Health. 2005. *Managing medicines in schools and early years settings.* London: DfES.

*within the scope of their employment. Local authorities may choose instead to 'self-insure' although in practice most do take out employer's liability insurance. Employers should make sure that their insurance arrangements provide full cover in respect of actions which could be taken by staff in the course of their employment. It is the employer's responsibility to ensure that proper procedures are in place and that staff are aware of the procedures and fully trained.*

Staff may be anxious about taking on responsibility for supporting children with complex health needs because they fear something 'going wrong'. In the event of a successful claim for alleged negligence it is the local authority or employer, not the employee who is held responsible and would meet the cost for damages, unless that member of staff has not followed their employer's policy.

### Training

Staff supporting children with complex health needs will require appropriate training and support from health professionals in order to carry out these tasks. The policy should outline the arrangements for the training of staff. Training is dealt with as a separate issue in chapter 7.

# 3 Anticipatory duties, planning and reasonable adjustments

Most children with complex health needs are likely to meet the definition of disability in the Disability Discrimination Act 1995 (DDA). This gives them protection from discrimination in a whole range of services. Social care, health care, and a range of services to the public, have been covered since the DDA was implemented in 1996. The SEN and Disability Act 2001 amended the DDA and extended its coverage to include education from September 2002.

Local authorities, health care agencies, schools and early education settings all have two key duties:
- not to treat disabled children 'less favourably'; and
- actively, to make 'reasonable adjustments' for disabled children.

The less favourable treatment duty means that services must not treat a disabled child less favourably than another child 'for a reason related to their disability' without justification. The most likely way in which a service might treat a disabled child less favourably is by having a blanket policy, for example:
- all children have to be toilet-trained before they come to this nursery'
- this school does not administer medicines. Parents are expected to come in and give their child any medicines their child needs during the school day'
- nursing staff are not permitted to lift or carry children

The reasonable adjustments duty requires services to think ahead, anticipate the barriers that disabled children may face and remove or minimise these barriers. The reasonable adjustments duty means that schools, services and settings need to have reviewed and, where necessary, made changes to their policies to ensure that they do not discriminate against disabled children. This might include re-arranging the school timetable, providing staff training, drafting new guidance for staff, or re-organising teaching areas to accommodate a child with a disability.

*Exemplar 4 (Daniel) highlights the issues raised for the school to ensure that Daniel could access his classrooms and the need for a height adjustable table in the science labs.*

Schools and LEAs are covered by Part IV of the DDA and must not discriminate in admissions, exclusions and 'education and associated services,' a term that covers every aspect of the life of the school. A *Code of practice*, published by the Disability Rights Commission provides guidance on the way that the duties operate. The code provides examples illustrating how the duties apply in practical situations in schools and LEAs. Ofsted expects to see evidence of practical adjustments being made in the classroom and in other areas of school life.

Under Part IV, if parents think that their child has been discriminated against, they have a right of redress by making a claim of disability discrimination to the SEN and Disability Tribunal. If the Tribunal finds that a school has discriminated unlawfully against a disabled pupil it can order any remedy that it sees fit, except financial compensation.

Schools and LEAs also have duties to prepare, review, revise if necessary and implement plans for improving accessibility for disabled pupils, over time. These plans must aim to increase participation in the curriculum, improve the physical environment of schools to increase access to the education and services provided, and improve the delivery of information to disabled pupils. As part of this duty, schools and LEAs should consider how they are improving links with services that can advise, support and train staff in increasing access to education and associated services for pupils with complex health needs.

Under Part III of the DDA, services and early years settings that are not constituted as schools (such as nurseries, family centres and pre-school provision, including playgroups and childminders) have duties not to discriminate by refusing to provide a service, offering a lower standard of service or offering a service on worse terms to a disabled child. Services and settings covered by Part III are not required to have accessibility plans, but, for them, the reasonable adjustments duty includes the requirement to provide auxiliary aids and services and to make physical alterations to buildings.

*Exemplar 3 (Anita) demonstrates the adjustments made by the nursery school to support Anita with her stoma care.*

Under Part III, if parents think that their child has been discriminated against, they have a right of redress by making a claim of disability discrimination through the county court. If the court finds that a service has discriminated unlawfully against a disabled child it can order any remedy that it sees fit, including financial compensation.

Further guidance on how the DDA applies to early years settings is available in *Early Years and the Disability Discrimination Act 1995 – what service providers need to know* available from the National Children's Bureau (020 7843 6000) or the Sure Start web site at www.surestart.gov.uk

Public bodies, including schools and local authorities will also have a duty, as a result of the Disability Discrimination Act 2005, to promote equality of opportunity for disabled people. Arrangements for supporting disabled children with complex health needs will be one aspect of this.

In order to carry out their duties to plan Bath and North East Somerset local authority have put in place the following arrangements:

*In January or February now each year a number of professionals (social services occupational therapists, NHS physiotherapists, SEN education officers, educational psychologists, school nurses, early years SENCOs and the schools capital organisation team) meet to identify new entrants to mainstream schools and those pupils who are transferring to junior or secondary schools, and who have complex medical needs.*

*This timing allows any additional physical adaptations to be made and staff trained as necessary. It also ensures that where additional support staff are needed they can be appointed and trained. The school nurses, lifetime nurses and local paediatricians continue to provide training in invasive medical techniques, etc as appropriate and support school staff. There is also support for pupils and staff from specialists such as the incontinence and diabetes nurses. In spite of this, the system is not yet perfect – there are always one or two children, unknown to any of the agencies, who appear at the last minute. The aim however is to ensure that every child starts school with the support that they need in place.*

Included at the end of this chapter is:

3.1 The audit information collated by Bath and North East Somerset local authority each year

## Disabled children entering schools in September 2004/5

| Name | Disability/ Medical condition | School | Adaptations |
|---|---|---|---|
| xxx Sept '04 | Downs Syndrome | xxx | Toilet handrails. Changing area. PT to check re incontinence with incontinence nurse. Will need full time LSA. SA to visit school Sept 2004   COMPLETE |
| xxx Sept '04 | Mobility | xxx | Toilet handrails   COMPLETE |
| xxx Sept '04 | Hemiplegia – reduced mobility – obese | xxx | Parents preferred school xxx. PT and SA to visit with family to check xxx's ability to move around school. Alternative school xxx   COMPLETE |
| xx Sept '04 | Epilepsy | xxx | Currently frequent grand mal episodes, but adjusting mediation. Trained LSA support needed   COMPLETE |
| xxx Sept '04 | Cerebral palsy | xxx | Completed ramp. LSA support and manual handling and hoist training needed.   COMPLETE |
| xxx Sept '04 | Mild Hemiplegia | xxx | Handrails on steps needed. NO STATEMENT. SA to check all OK Sept 2004.   COMPLETE |
| xxx Sept '04 | Pulmonary Hypertension | xxx | Life threatening – Lifetime Nurse involved. Storage for O2 cylinders; LSA & manual handling training needed. COMPLETE |
| xxx Sept '04 | Autistic Spectrum | xxx | Playground safety. Washing/changing facilities. PT to check if he is a runner/ toilet training. Additional accessible toilet needed, would have to be new build.   COMPLETE |
| xxx Sept '04 | Hemiplegia | xxx | Walks very well. Should have no problems.   COMPLETE |

| Name | Disability/ Medical condition | School | Adaptations |
|------|------|------|------|
| xxx Sept '05 | Complex cerebral palsy | xxx | Bright electric wheelchair user. OT to visit with pupil/parents. SA will need to visit school after discussion with OT. Possibly ramps, handrails hoist needed. LSA training in manual handling and use of hoist. |
| xxx Sept '05 | Autistic | xxx | Not toilet trained |
| xxx Sept '05 | Cerebral palsy | xxx | Walks with frame SA to visit with OT and pupils/parents April 2004. COMPLETE |
| xxx Sept '05 | Achondroplasia | xxx | Probably OK. SA to visit with parents/ pupil April 2005. |
| xxx Sept '05 | Downs Syndrome | xxx | No apparent problems. SA to check April '05.   COMPLETE |
| xxx Sept '05 | Mild Diaplegia | xxx | No apparent problems. SA to check April '05.   COMPLETE |
| xxx Sept '05 | Degenerative condition. Trembles, fits | xxx | LSA support |
| xxx Sept '05 | Mild hemiplegia | xxx | No apparent problems. SA to check April '05.   COMPLETE |
| xxx Sept '05 | Diplegia | xxx | Walking but very wobbly, 1:1 support No apparent problems. SA to check April '05.   COMPLETE |
| xxx Sept '05 | Deaf (cochlea implants) Low muscle tone | xxx | Walking difficulties cannot manage steps/ramps. May need to suggest alternative school. SA to check April '05. COMPLETE |
| xxx Sept '05 | Deaf + physical disabilities | xxx | SA to talk to Bristol City OT and visit school. |

# 4 Admissions

Children with complex health needs have the same rights of admission to a school or setting as other children. During the admissions process, schools and other settings should take the opportunity to collect information from parents which will assist in developing the best possible support for each child with complex health needs.

The process of admission, particularly the period prior to admission, is crucial in collecting information about the child, identifying potential risks and identifying the specific areas in which staff will require training from health professionals

In order to ensure the smooth transfer from one school or early years setting to the next, schools should be informed about complex health needs, well in advance. Meeting the needs of children with complex health needs may require time to plan and make reasonable adjustments or to put into place support arrangements. An example of an 'Admissions Form' which would identify children with complex health needs in a mainstream setting can be found at the end of this chapter.

**example** The following issues are included on a checklist for schools devised by Hackney Learning Trust and the City and Hackney Teaching Primary Care Trust:

- How will the child get to school?
- How will the child get around the building, into classrooms, toilets?
- What issues arise for school outings?
- Will quiet distraction free workspaces and/or dinner times be necessary and available?
- At what level are the child's self help skills including eating, drinking, toileting?
- What equipment will be needed? Eg. toiletting equipment, nappy disposal, standing frames, technology.
- Does the child have medical needs?
- What issues arise for the child at play times and lunch eg. Friends, equipment, not coping with noise in the dinner hall?
- How will the child access curriculum levels? Notify curriculum coordinators in relation to planning and providing resources.
- Does the child need adult support – in the classroom, at lunch, at play time, around the school?
- What additional skills will adults need in relation to learning, social and

*emotional, physical and medical needs? What is the plan for training the staff?*

- *How many additional people will need to be trained if the child needs assistance with feeding or toileting?*
- *What preparation is necessary for all staff, children and parents before this child starts?*

Local authorities and other employers may produce general information on particular conditions. It is important that this information should give staff an understanding about a particular condition as well as how that condition is likely to affect the child in a school or early years setting. This type of information should not be seen to replace training which staff may require or information about an individual child's particular needs provided by a health professional.

Information sheets tend to cover the most common conditions. Staff can also find additional information on various websites. Most national organisations supporting individuals with a specific condition have websites which will give general information about a particular condition.

Contact a Family is a national organisation which operates an advice helpline, as well, as producing a directory of rare conditions. Their contact details are listed in the Resource section at the end of this handbook. The Early Support Programme also has a range of publications about specific conditions as they apply to children in the pre-school age range (see www.earlysupport.org.uk).

*Exemplar 3 (Anita) highlights the use the nursery made of literature produced by the National Advisory Service for Parents of Children with a Stoma.*

### Information sharing

Parents and carers have prime responsibility for their children's health and they should inform the school or early years setting about any health needs. However, there is no requirement on them to do so, and parents may decide not to tell the school or setting about a particular condition. The school or early years setting therefore needs to take a proactive role: asking parents about their child's needs, promoting an atmosphere which is open and in which parents feel comfortable to disclose information, safe in the knowledge that such information:

- will not be used to bar their child from the school or setting, or from activities within the school or setting;
- will be used sensitively to help their child make the most of their time in school or setting;
- will be communicated to staff who need to know what reasonable adjustments should be made for their child.

## Confidentiality

The Disability Discrimination Act says that, in deciding what sort of reasonable adjustments to make, a school must take into account a request for confidentiality as to the nature or the existence of a child's disability:
- from the child's parents; and
- from the child, if the school is satisfied that the child understands the nature and the effect of the request for confidentiality.

The legislation recognises that a request for confidentiality may limit the reasonable adjustments that a school can make. The child's safety will always be the first consideration. If a request for confidentiality meant that staff taking pupils on a trip could not be informed of the nature of a child's condition, and if ignorance of the child's condition could put the child at risk, the school might not be able to include the pupil on that trip.

In practice, the very reasons that parents may request confidentiality relate back to concerns that information might not be used sensitively to support their child, or that their child might be singled out in some way. Parents' concerns are likely to be heightened where there is a social stigma attached to the child's health condition.

It comes back to the same principle as above: if parents are confident that information that they share with the school will be handled sensitively, parents are more likely to share that information with the school in the first place and less likely to request confidentiality if they do share it.

Whilst the DDA applies these duties to schools, the same principles apply to early years settings.

*Exemplar 5 (Bethan) illustrates good practice with regard to information sharing and confidentiality.*

Included at the end of this chapter are:
4.1 The pastoral care and admission form used by Walton Girls' High School
4.2 The DDA form used by Walton Girls' High School

## Confidential
*Please see the attached completion notes.*

## Pupil details

Pupil's legal surname _____

Pupil's surname _____
*(if different from legal surname)*

Forenames _____
*(underline the name used)*

Date of birth _____

## Parents/guardians/carers:
*(delete as appropriate)*

Mr and Mrs/Mr/Mrs/Miss/Ms/other _____
*(correspondence will be addressed to the above)*

Relationship to pupil _____

Address _____

_____

Post code _____

Home telephone _____

## Emergency contacts

*First contact name* _____

Relationship _____ Telephone _____

Ask for _____ Location _____

*Second contact name* _____

Relationship _____ Telephone _____

Ask for _____ Location _____

*Third contact name* _____

Relationship _____ Telephone _____

Ask for _____ Location _____

## Details of parent: if separated

Name _____

Address _____

_____

Post code _____

*Please tick if a second report is required to be sent to this address* ☐

## Schooling details

Name of previous school _____

County/Education Authority _____

Town _____

## Name(s) of sister(s) who are attending, or have attended Walton

Child in public care ☐ yes ☐ no

Authority _____

## Religion

☐ Hindu ☐ Jewish ☐ Christian ☐ Sikh

☐ Muslim ☐ No religion ☐ Other, details _____

## Home language _____

## Second language _____

## Medical information

Doctor's name _____

Surgery _____

Telephone _____

## Medical details

Does your daughter have:

1 any health condition or disability? ☐ yes ☐ no

2 Has it lasted or is it expected to last 12 months? ☐ yes ☐ no

3 Does this have an adverse effect on your daughter's
  day to day activities? ☐ yes ☐ no

*If you have answered yes to all of the three questions please ask for a Disability Discrimination Act form which will enable us to identify what we need to do to support your daughter at school.*

Does your daughter:

- have any medical condition? (eg diabetes) ☐ yes ☐ no
- take regular medication? ☐ yes ☐ no
- suffer from impaired hearing? ☐ yes ☐ no
- use an inhaler? ☐ yes ☐ no
- not suffer from any allergy? ☐ yes ☐ no
- wear glasses? ☐ yes ☐ no

*If you have answered yes to any of the above questions please give further information*

**Parents are requested to read the statement below and then sign and date this form**

☐ I/we received a copy of the school brochure and agree to support the school by encouraging my/our daughter to abide by the discipline procedures and code of conduct contained within.

☐ I agree to my daughter's photograph being used for school promotions.
*(Please see separate letter)*

*(please tick)*

Parent's signature _____
*Mother/father/guardian/carer – please delete as appropriate*

Date _____

# The DDA form used by Walton Girls' High School

**Student name** _____

**Date of birth** _____

1 Does your daughter have any health condition or disability?  ☐ yes  ☐ no

2 Has it lasted or is it expected to last 12 months?  ☐ yes  ☐ no

3 Does this have an adverse effect on your daughter's day-to-day activities?  ☐ yes  ☐ no

*If you have answered yes to all three questions your daughter is likely to have met the DDA definition of disabled. If so, please tick the boxes below that most accurately describe your daughter health condition or disability. The information will help us to identify what we need to do to support your daughter at school.*

Does/will your daughter have difficulty with:

1 Moving about the school and going on school visits  ☐ yes  ☐ no

2 Use of hands and fingers (eg to hold a pen or pencil)  ☐ yes  ☐ no

3 Lifting, carrying or moving objects (eg carrying school bag)  ☐ yes  ☐ no

4 Washing, going to the toilet, controlling the need to go to the toilet, dressing, etc  ☐ yes  ☐ no

5 Expressing herself or understanding what others are saying  ☐ yes  ☐ no

6 All of the work in school including reading, writing, number work or understanding information  ☐ yes  ☐ no

7 Hearing or eyesight  ☐ yes  ☐ no

8 Making friends, relating to adults, behaving properly in school  ☐ yes  ☐ no

9 A medical need which has lasted or is expected to last more than 12 months and takes regular medication *(please give details under any other information)*  ☐ yes  ☐ no

10 Complex health needs requiring daily assistance in order to maintain optimum health such as physiotherapy at school  ☐ yes  ☐ no

Any other information we need to know about your daughter's disability

_____

_____

Parent's signature _____

Date _____

# 5 Risk management and assessment

There is an element of risk involved with many of the tasks carried out to support children with complex health needs. These risks cannot be removed completely, but it is possible to manage them. Risk management will form the basis of ensuring that children with complex health needs are included in schools and early years settings.

Risk management should cover activities which take place both on site as well as activities which take place 'off-site', such as educational visits and trips.

For staff, risk management will ensure:
- that tasks are carried out in the safest possible way
- that any risk to staff is minimised

For children, risk management with ensure:
- that they are not exposed to unacceptable risks
- that they can take part and enjoy all the activities of the school or early years setting

### The elements in risk management
- **Risk** refers to the possibility of a situation occurring which would involve exposure to danger or a hazard, that is, the possibility of something harmful happening.
- Risk is a combination of the **likelihood** of something harmful happening and the **seriousness** of the potential injury.
- A hazard is less likely to cause harm if certain **controls** are in place. Controls are the steps taken either to eliminate the hazard or reduce the associated risk to an acceptably low level.
- Risk is managed by **assessing it**, avoiding it if it is unnecessary or reducing it to a level which is 'reasonably practicable'.
- When considering what is '**reasonably practicable**' the needs of both the child and staff should be taken into account.
- **Reasonably practicable**, as defined by the Health and Safety Executive (HSE), means *'an employee has satisfied his/her duty if he/she can show that any further preventative steps would be grossly disproportionate to the further benefit which would accrue from their introduction'*. (HSE 1992, p 8)
- A key element in any risk management strategy is child protection. Risk assessments should cover issues relating to child protection, for example, intimate care that may be required when carrying out a

procedure for a particular child. The assessment should balance both the child's right to kept safe with the right to be treated with dignity

In order to manage risk, schools and early years settings will need to:
- clarify who is responsible for carrying out risk assessments
- detail the training required to carry out risk assessments
- develop the procedures and paperwork required to carrying out risk assessments
- agree on arrangements to monitor and review all risk assessments on a regular basis

### 'Think safety'

Many local authorities employ health and safety officers to carry out risk assessments, and whilst their role and specialism is vital, all staff working with children should have an awareness of health and safety issues and how to assess and minimise risk.

Good practice in this area of work indicates that risk assessment and risk management should not rely solely on health and safety officers. Assessments and policies should be written in a way that all staff can understand them. The forms and how to assess a new situation should be written in plain English rather than in health and safety jargon.

Training staff in risk management is about training staff to think 'safety' rather than training staff to complete risk assessment forms. This will mean, whatever situation staff find themselves in, they will feel confident at looking at the situation and identifying the potential risks.

### The general and the specific

Risk assessments will cover general situations as well as situations and tasks which are specific to each child and each procedure. It is usually during the process of admitting a child to a new school or early years setting that the risks specific to that child need to be identified. An individual health care plan can help staff identify additional needs of a child and clarify the safety measures which need to be in place.

### Addressing fears about managing risk

Staff may have a number of concerns about the risks involved to both children and staff in ensuring the inclusion of children with complex health needs in mainstream settings, including the fear that they will be blamed if something goes wrong, lack of insurance, inadequate training. These anxieties can be minimised if staff assess all relevant areas of risk, take adequate steps to minimise them and ensure that their actions are 'reasonably practicable'. Insurance and training are covered elsewhere in this handbook.

### Moving and handling

Many children with complex health needs use wheelchairs or need additional assistance in terms of moving around. Moving and handling should form part of the risk management plan for such children. As with other risk assessments, assessments on moving and handling are likely to be both general (eg. applicable to all the children who use wheelchairs) as well as specific (relate to the particular needs of an individual child). Occupational Therapists and Physiotherapists will be able to offer expertise with regard to equipment children may need.

*Exemplar 4 (Daniel) highlights the type of issues likely to arise from the risk assessments for a child who uses a wheelchair.*

There is specific legislation and guidance which covers the management of risk in this area. The regulations state that risk assessments should cover:
- the lifting task: why is it required, are there alternatives
- the child or young person's weight, needs and abilities
- the physical environment
- the individual capacity of the person doing the lifting

Further information on this legislation is detailed in Appendix 2.

### Specific policies

In addition to moving and handling, there are other areas which have specific regulations and guidance and they are likely to be covered in the employer's health and safety policy and guidance. These areas are:
- storage of medicines
- Control of Substances Hazardous to Health regulations 2002 (COSHH)
- clinical waste
- infection control
- fire and evacuation procedures

*All the exemplars demonstrate the importance of these specific policies.*

Included at the end of this chapter are:
5.1 A medical needs risk assessment from Bath and North East Somerset local authority
5.2 A risk assessment for two children with brittle bones from the Learning Trust in Hackney
5.3 Manual handling assessment from Nottinghamshire Education Authority. This assessment is carried out by a safe handling advisor together with the parent, child and support assistant who will be working with the child. The form details the risks and controls and also gives detailed instructions on each move or lift required by the child. (There are separate instructions for hoisting not covered on the form.) Each assessment has a manual handling care plan which is a summary of the whole situation and staff can see at a glance if equipment is on order or when the plan needs to be reviewed.

Date __January 2004__

School _____

Pupil _____

Age __5 years__

Medical condition Pulmonary Hypertension

| List significant hazards | Who is at risk? | List existing controls | List additional controls necessary | Date for completion | Date completed |
|---|---|---|---|---|---|
| Life threatening medical condition | xxx | Lifetime Nurse discussions with xxx's teacher and other key staff. | Resuscitation training for xxx's LSAs | ASAP | |
| | | Emergency procedure agreed with lifetime nurse and all staff informed. First aiders always available during school hours. | Regular review with lifetime nurse – termly in first instance | April '04 | |
| | | xxx's mother is the only person to attend to the Hickman line and oxygen cylinder until LSAs are trained and competent. | LSA training by lifetime nurse | January '04 | |
| Hickman line and pump could be dislodged due to lack of care by other children in reception class and at playtime. | xxx | All pupils informed during assembly of xxx's need to wear the pump to save her life, not to tamper with it and to avoid bumping into her, etc. | Supervision at all times | Ongoing | |
| Access to oxygen cylinder required at all times so hazard of: 1 storage 2 handling 3 transportation | xxx/staff/ pupils | Oxygen only in school when xxxxxx is present. Only mini cylinders used which her mother transports to school in a pushchair and handles in the classroom, where it is locked in the teacher's cupboard, away from heat/electrical sources. (As agreed with the lifetime nurse/health & safety) | | | |

Assessor _____

Reassessment due __April 2004__

## Risk assessment

Name _____

School _____

Date of birth _____

Condition  Brittle bones

*Information*  Susceptible to fractures. Care and attention should be paid to any movement in and around school. The pupil may tire easily, especially on school journeys or visits. All staff must be aware of the pupil's needs and this care plan. Consider whether the adult should hold the pupil's hand at all times of transition.

| *Activity* | *Risk* | *Supervision* | *Additional comments* |
|---|---|---|---|
| Arrival and departure from school | Tripping, falling or impact with other pupils | Parents/carers | If parents/carers are unable to bring child to and from the classroom they will liaise with the class teacher to make suitable arrangements |
| Class activities | Small classroom – risk of: injury by bumping, falling, movement of furniture eg chair or tables | Class teacher and teaching assistant (TA) | • Careful classroom organisation<br>• Primary pupil should sit on a chair for carpet time |
| PE and games lessons (including changing) | Potentially higher risk activities | Class teacher – lesson planning. TA to support throughout the session | Individual needs to be incorporated into all lesson plans. Advice must be sought from the school or specialist nurse and the occupational therapist |
| Break times (including movement to and from the classroom) | Tripping, falling or impact with other pupils | TA to cover morning break and afternoon break (where there is one) | • TA to supervise from and return to the classroom<br>• At lunchtimes this will entail movement from classroom to dining hall back to the playground and return to the classroom<br>• If the weather is cold or wet the pupil should remain inside in a pre-arranged place<br>• It is often helpful to invite another pupil, who may be a friend, to remain inside with the pupil |
| Lunch | Tripping, falling, impact with other pupils, furniture or trays, etc | Classteacher and TA | TA to supervise the movement from classroom to the dining hall.<br>Also see above |

| Activity | Risk | Supervision | Additional comments |
|---|---|---|---|
| Toileting | Tripping, falling or impact with other pupils | TA or parent | Parent/carer to ensure the child has visited the toilet before the start of school. TA should ensure visits to the toilet at break and lunch times. The pupil must be escorted. During lesson times the class teacher or TA will make decisions about who escorts the pupil |
| School visits | Higher risk. Tripping, falling or impact with other pupils or obstacles. Tiring quickly if it is a strenuous or long day | Parent and class teacher | The trip must be planned in advance taking into account the pupil's needs, particularly transport. TLT has produced some guidance on this. A 'taxi card' may be helpful. Advice can be sought from TLT Manager for Inclusion or the Health and Safety Officer |
| Emergency procedures | High risk | Class teacher or TA. The class teacher has overall responsibility | Pupil should follow with an adult at the back of the class group or with the class teacher if there is no other adult available. Advice should be sought from the fire service |
| Information sharing | High risk A new adult in the classroom without prior knowledge or familiarity with the pupil's needs | Class teacher and SENCO. Headteacher ensures all staff are adequately informed. There must be a procedure for training and delegation | Information sheet and any care plans must be available for any new adult working in the classroom |
| Site specific information | Eg The school is built over a number of different levels with many staircases. | Class teacher | Movement around the building during the school day must be carefully considered and planned for |

Date plan agreed _____     Review date _____

Plan agreed by:
parent or carer _____

SENCO _____

pupil _____

TA _____

class teacher _____
*(additional people should insert their designation)*

The review period should not be extended beyond a year but can be reduced, eg termly, if required

# Manual handling assessment from Nottinghamshire Education Authority

## Nottinghamshire LEA manual handling form IPA 1

### Individual pupil assessment

Name  Jane Smith

Date of birth _____  Class _____

Male/female  Female  Weight/build  Medium

Condition  Cerebral Palsy

| | Abilities | Equipment normally used |
|---|---|---|
| Communication | | |
| Walking | 1 carer assisted | Handling belt |
| Standing/sitting | 1 carer assisted | Chair/table to lean on |
| Personal care | 1 carer assisted | Toilet step   Hand rails |
| Transfers | To/from power chair | |

| | | Yes | Notes |
|---|---|---|---|
| 1 | Does weight/size/shape of pupil present risk? | * | Jane is growing rapidly Her level of stability is unpredictable |
| 2 | Does communication present a risk? | | |
| 3 | Does comprehension present a risk? | | |
| 4 | Is there a history of falls? | | |
| 5 | Are there medical considerations? | * | Hips prone to dislocation |
| 6 | Is pain/discomfort a risk factor? | | |
| 7 | Do clothes/equipment/appliances present a risk? | | |
| 8 | Does behaviour present a risk? | * | Jane performs better when she has an 'audience'. Her level of stability is unpredictable |
| 9 | Is frequency of handling a risk? | * | Same carer for most transfers Repetitive tasks |
| 10 | Insufficient rest or recovery periods | * | Same carer for most transfers |
| 11 | Do attitudes/feelings present a risk | | |
| 12 | Are there any environmental risks? | | |
| 13. | Are there risks concerning individual capability (child) | | |
| 14 | Are there risks concerning individual capability (staff) | * | 1 carer – back injury 1 carer – history of knee injury |

## Risks identified and action plan

| Risk identified | Action plan | Date of completion |
|---|---|---|
| 1 Jane is growing rapidly Her level of stability is unpredictable. | Staff to be aware of changes occurring. | |
| 5 Hips prone to dislocation. | Staff awareness. | |
| 8 Jane performs better when she has an 'audience'. Her level of stability is unpredictable | Staff/therapist/assessor awareness! Staff to use own judgement re Jane's ability/willingness to assist. | |
| 9 Same carer for most transfers Repetitive tasks | Reduce number of supported standing sessions. | |
| 10 Same carer for most transfers | Minimise manual handling where possible (as above). | |
| 14 1 carer – back injury 1 carer – history of knee injury | Staff to be aware of own capabilities. | |

### *Safe system of work*

Nottinghamshire LEA's manual handling policy, in accordance with MHO Regs 1992, states that carers following this safe system of work must hold a current manual handling certificate and have received instruction in the use of all relevant equipment

*Carers should take responsibility for their own postures and personal safety throughout all manual handling procedures*

### Carers' instructions

- **Standing/sitting (from class chair)** *1 carer to assist*

  Carer sits at the side of Jane's chair on wheeled stool or box. Carer steadies chair by holding chair legs. Jane moves herself to stand/sit (nose over toes). Jane's standing is extremely slow and controlled. Patience and verbal prompts are required.

- **Supported standing** *1 carer to assist*

  Encourage Jane to stand – as above. Carer sits behind Jane on a low wooden box. Position hands on Jane's knees to provide support (flat palms) and pull knees slightly back to maintain straight legs. The left knee also needs to be pulled slightly towards the centre. This will enable Jane to stand with straight legs and feet flat on the floor (but affects her upper body control.)

  *or*

  Encourage Jane to stand – as above. Carer sits behind Jane on a low wooden box. Position hands on Jane's hips to provide support at the pelvis. This will enable Jane to stand upright with hips facing forwards (but her legs are not straight nor her feet correctly planted).

  Carers to alternate between the above techniques.

  *Jane is required to stand for periods not exceeding 10 minutes.*

*Including me*

- **Assisted walking** *1 carer to assist*

  Jane walks with support from a carer walking upright behind her. Carer holds her right hand with left palm on Jane's back for support/reassurance.

  *or*

  Jane wears a handling belt and a carer sits behind her on wheeled stool to provide support.

- **Toiletting** *1 carer to assist*

  Jane enters the toilet in her power chair. Carer to remove footplates and position foot box/step in front of toilet. Position w/ch alongside washbasin in front of the toilet and guide Jane's feet onto box step. Carer to position drop down rail and assist Jane to stand from her w/ch – supporting at left elbow or hand, and right hip if necessary. Encourage Jane to hold onto horizontal rail on the right as she turns. Carer to raise drop down rail to create space. Carer adjusts Jane's clothing at this point.  then lowers herself to sit on the toilet – releasing her hold on the horizontal rail and sometimes holding the vertical. Carer again needs to lower the drop down rail. Leave the wheelchair in position. Carer to leave cubicle and wait outside – Jane will call when she needs assistance.

  Reverse above. After adjusting Jane's clothing assist her to turn and sit down into w/ch.

  Jane washes her hands once seated in her w/ch.

  *Jane requires verbal prompts throughout to ensure good positioning of her hands and feet. It is essential that she is afforded sufficient time to complete this transfer as independently as possible. Patience is, therefore, required.*

- **Out of power chair** *1 carer to assist*

  Carer folds footplates to the side. Jane adjusts her position, moving forward in the chair until her feet touch the floor. Carer to stand at an oblique angle slightly forward of Jane, to prevent falls. Carer to support Jane to relevant piece of equipment/location.

- **Into power chair** *1 carer to assist*

  Jane walks to her w/ch. She turns and backs up until her bottom is touching the wheelchair seat cushion. Jane needs to be encouraged/reminded to push through her knees to maintain her stability. Carer kneels to reposition one footplate. Carer to guide Jane's foot onto the footplate (verbal and physical prompts required at this point). Encourage Jane to push up and back. Once she is safely seated carer to reposition second footplate. Again ask Jane to push up and back to attain a good sitting position – fine tune if necessary.

| | | | | |
|---|---|---|---|---|
| Date assessed | *October 2004* | | | |
| Assessor's signature | | | | |
| TA signature | | | | |
| Pupil signature | | | | |
| Proposed review dates | *April 2005 or as requested* | | | |

## Manual handling care plan

Name of pupil _____

DOB _____ Build _____

Name of assessor _____

### Handling constraints relating to disability, medical condition, comprehension, behaviour, co-operation

Can weight bear and is co-operative – but her ability is variable. She needs verbal support and encouragement.

### Degree of independence, mobility/weight bearing ability, likelihood of falls, etc

Danger of falling if unsupervised/unfocused.

| Tasks (see examples) | Methods to be used (see examples) Consult standard protocols for more detailed description | Remaining problems and further measures required (see examples) |
|---|---|---|
| Assisted walking | 1 carer<br>Handling belt<br>Wheeled stool | |
| Class stool/chair | Minimum 1 carer assisted | |
| Standing/sitting | Minimum 1 carer assisted | |
| Toiletting | Minimum 1 carer assisted<br>Footblock<br>Grab rails | |
| In/out of wheelchair | Minimum 1 carer assisted | |

| | | | | |
|---|---|---|---|---|
| Date assessed | _October 2004_ | _____ | _____ | _____ |
| Assessor's signature | _____ | _____ | _____ | _____ |
| TA signature | _____ | _____ | _____ | _____ |
| Pupil signature | _____ | _____ | _____ | _____ |
| Proposed review dates | _April 2005 or as requested_ | _____ | _____ | _____ |

### Check list

**Tasks**

| | |
|---|---|
| Sitting/standing | * |
| Toiletting | * |
| Walking | * |
| Transfer to standing frame | |
| Movement on bed or plinth | |
| PE swimming hydrotherapy | |
| Washing and bathing | |
| Floor | * |
| Arrival/departure | |

**Methods to be used**

| | |
|---|---|
| Hoist | |
| Standing hoist | |
| Bath hoist | |
| Number of staff | 1 |
| Specific room | * |
| Slings | |
| Changing bed/plinth | |
| Wheeled sani chair | |
| Turntable | |
| Sliding aids | |
| Grabrails | * |
| Stair lift | |

**Remaining problems and further measures required**

| | |
|---|---|
| Medical condition eg spasm/stiffness | * |
| Changes to layout or furniture | |
| Change of route | |
| Training | |
| Medical issue with carer, eg pregnant/back problem | * |

# 6 Health care plans

Children with complex health needs should have health care plans. Each child should have an individual plan which is specific to their particular needs. Plans will vary in length and complexity, depending on the needs of a particular child. Health care plans will be read and used by a range of staff so they should be written in non-jargon, non-medical language which is easy to understand. Where children take medicines the health care plan should cover medicines as well as other forms of support required.

## Why are health care plans necessary?

A health care plan is important because it clarifies:
- for staff, parents and children the level of support a child will receive in any setting
- who is responsible for each task or procedure relating to a particular child
- the training required for particular procedures and who will carry out the training

## What should a health care plan cover?

A health care plan should adopt a holistic approach detailing all aspects of the child's condition, as well as the medicines and support required and set out:
- particular procedures that should be carried out, including who should carry out those procedures and the training they can expect
- protocols for exchanging information between agencies (with clearly defined lines of responsibility and named contacts)
- additional risk assessments required for that particular child – who is responsible for carrying them out
- any special health care needs with may affect the child's use of services such as transport or play activities, implementation of therapy programmes, etc
- the use, storage and maintenance of any equipment
- any arrangements for the provision of education or associated services when the child is too unwell to attend school or is in hospital or another health care setting
- parental wishes for the child
- information on the manner in which the child prefers any task to be carried out, in order to ensure consistency of approach across all settings the child attends
- any anticipated changes in the child's condition or care routine
- arrangements for reviewing the plan

### How should a health care plan be drawn up?

- Prior to the child starting at a school or another setting a meeting should be held to draw up the health care plan
- The purpose of the meeting is to identify the child's needs and draw up a plan which will support the child in that setting
- All individuals who hold key information on the child should be invited to contribute to the meeting. The meeting should be multi-agency
- Parents and where appropriate, the child (depending on the age and understanding of the child) should be invited to take part in drawing up the health care plan
- The plan should be agreed by the various agencies who have contributed, and signed by the parents
- Health care plans should be 'live documents which can be altered, in writing if the child's needs change. There should be agreement as to who can alter the plan. Changes to health procedures or medicines would need to be made by the appropriate health care professional.
- The health care plan should be regularly reviewed. If a child has a statement of special educational needs, the health care plan should be reviewed at the time of the annual review or more frequently if the child's needs change.

*All the exemplars highlight the importance of a planning meeting prior to the child attending school or when the needs of the child change.*

Details of drawing up a health care plan are outlined in *Managing medicines in schools and early years settings* (DfES/DH, 2005). A copy of the health care plan is included at the end of this chapter.

### Agreeing health care plans across all agencies

In North Yorkshire, the Scarborough, Whitby and Rydale health trust has led an initiative to develop health care plans for children with medical needs and those with complex health needs. These plans are agreed and used consistently across all agencies – health, education, social services and the voluntary sector. The health care plan for complex needs is included at the end of this chapter.

### Access to the health care plan

The health care plan should be kept in a place which is accessible to staff, but which takes into account the need for confidentiality. This may mean that protocols for dealing with emergencies are referred to in the health care plan but are kept in a place which can be accessed in an emergency.

> Included at the end of this chapter are:
> 6.1 Health care plan – 'Managing medicines in schools and early years settings' (DfES/DH, 2005)
> 6.2 Health care plan for complex health needs from Scarborough, Whitby and Ryedale Primary Care Trust

# Health care plan – 'Managing medicines in schools and early years settings' (DIES/DH, 2005)

Name of school/setting _____

Child's name _____

Group/class/form _____ Date of birth _____

Child's address _____

_____

Medical diagnosis or condition _____

Date _____ Review date _____

**Family contact information**

Name _____

Phone (work) _____ (home) _____ (mobile) _____

Name _____

Phone (work) _____ (home) _____ (mobile) _____

**Clinic/hospital contact**

Name _____ Phone _____

**GP**

Name _____ Phone _____

Describe medical needs and give details of child's symptoms

_____

Daily care requirements *(eg before sport/at lunchtime)*

_____

Describe what constitutes an emergency for the child, and the action to take if this occurs

_____

Follow up care

_____

Who is responsible in an emergency (state if different for off-site activities)

_____

Form copied to

_____

Level 2

## HEALTH CARE PLAN
## COMPLEX MEDICAL NEEDS

Name of child/young person _____

D.O.B _____

Home address _____

_____

Telephone _____

Hospital number or NHS number _____

School/nursery _____

Telephone _____

Parents/carers _____

Relationship to child/young person _____

Address _____

_____

Telephone  Home _____  Work _____

Mobile _____

Parental responsibility _____

Alternative emergency contact _____

Relationship _____

Address _____

_____

Telephone _____

Completed date _____

photograph

Consultant/hospital contact _____

Address _____

_____ Telephone _____

GP name _____

Address _____

_____ Telephone _____

Community paediatrician _____

Address _____

_____ Telephone _____

Health visitor/school nurse _____

Address _____

_____ Telephone _____

Community children's nurse _____

Address _____

_____ Telephone _____

Therapist _____

Address _____

_____ Telephone _____

Dietitian _____

Address _____

_____ Telephone _____

Care manager (Social services) _____

Address _____

_____ Telephone _____

Project manager (NCH) _____

Address _____

_____ Telephone _____

Description of clinical condition

_____

_____

_____

Description of daily care needs to include as applicable: equipment, continence care, medication, allergies, behavioural needs.

_____

_____

_____

Description of what constitutes an emergency (signs, symptoms, etc.) and the action to be taken.

_____

_____

_____

Additional plan in place *(eg Epipen, Rectal Diazepam, Midazolam)*     yes/no

_____

_____

_____

Who has responsibility in an emergency? _____

Nominated adult who has received training. _____

This healthcare plan completed by

Signature _____ Date _____

Healthcare plan agreed by

Name _____

Designation _____

Signature _____ Date _____

Authorised person/s trained to undertake clinical procedure _____

Adults who have received appropriate training identified in central register.

Name _____

Signature _____ Date _____

Name _____

Signature _____ Date _____

Name _____

Signature _____ Date _____

Name _____

Signature _____ Date _____

Care manager/project manager

Name _____

Signature _____ Date _____

Headteacher

Name _____

Signature _____ Date _____

## Parental/guardian consent

I consent to staff named above/carer administering these procedures for my child, and I consent to the information in this healthcare plan being shared with non-parent carers.

Name _____

Relationship to child/young person _____

Signature _____ Date _____

## Child's consent *(wherever possible)*

I consent to staff/carer administering the above procedure to me.

Signature _____ Date _____

Copies held by _____

Notification of any changes will be made by _____

# 7 Training of staff

Training of staff is an integral part of any policy on managing complex health needs.

### Clinical procedures which might be undertaken by non-health qualified staff

In supporting children with complex health needs in schools and early years settings there are a number of clinical procedures which staff may be trained to undertake. In the main such training is undertaken by nursing staff, usually school nurses or community children's nurses who are employed by primary care trusts or other NHS trusts. The Royal College of Nursing has provided the following advisory list of procedures which may be safely taught and delegated to non-health qualified staff (agreed as of June 2005).

- administering prescribed medicine in pre-measured dose via nasogastric tube or gastrostomy tube
- bolus or continuous feeds via a nasogastric or gastrostomy tube
- tracheostomy care including suction and emergency change of tracheostomy tube
- injections (intramusculuar or subcutaneous) with pre-loaded syringe
- intermittent catheterisation and catheter care
- care of a Mitrofanoff
- stoma care
- inserting suppositories or pessaries with a pre-packaged dose of a prescribed medicine
- rectal medication with a pre-packaged dose
- administration of buccal or intra-nasal Midazolam
- emergency treatments covered in basic first aid training
- assistance with inhalers, insufflation cartridges and nebulisers
- assistance with oxygen administration
- basic life support/resuscitation

The Royal College of Nursing has also advised that the following tasks should not be undertaken by non-health qualified carers

- re-insertion of nasogastric tube
- re-insertion of gastrostomy tube
- injections involving: assembling syringe, administering intravenously or controlled drugs.
- programming of syringe drivers
- filling of oxygen cylinders

These lists are provided here as a general guide only and it is important to acknowledge that for children with complex health needs creative and innovative solutions are sometimes required. However, it is absolutely imperative that any delegation of clinical tasks to non-health qualified staff is undertaken within a robust governance framework an integral part of which will be the arrangement for:
- initial training and preparation of staff
- assessment and confirmation of competence of staff
- confirmation of arrangements for on-going support, updating of training and re-assessment of competence of staff

Training should take place at two levels:
- general training around complex health needs
- training around a specific child and the procedures or care that child will require

In the same way as information is shared on a need-to-know basis, training should be arranged on a general level for all staff working with a particular child and specific training for staff who support a child on a one-to-one basis.

*The exemplars demonstrate good practice with regard to training at both a general and specific level.*

## Management of training

The way in which training is arranged and delivered will vary from one area to another. This chapter will look at two examples of how training may be organised and delivered. The examples draw on good practice from different parts of the country.

**Birmingham**, one of the largest local authorities in England and currently has four primary care trusts. The training of staff is organised and delivered by one of the primary care trusts on behalf of the others. The example below details the work undertaken by the South Birmingham Primary Care NHS trust, Children's Services Directorate. At present this arrangement only covers the 500 local education authority schools in the area.

*In 1995 through joint health and education funding two nurse advisors were appointed to support children with medical needs in schools. This was initially a pilot scheme. Due to the success of the pilot and the drive towards inclusion these posts became permanent in 1998. The team was expanded in 2004 to include to part-time nurse educators.*

*The team have a number of roles:*
- *advice around medical needs to the local education authority*
- *training, advice and support to schools – delivery of approximately 400 training sessions a year*

- training, advice and support to primary health care staff. They do not replace the role of the school nurses, but provide specialist advice and support when required
- offer advice to and take direct referrals from specialist health staff, for example, paediatric consultants
- provide advice for national specialist organisations and other PCTs
- offer advice and support to parents, children and young people

The work of the team includes:
- development of local medical needs guidance for schools – each school has been issued with a school health folder to store relevant information that they will need to manage health needs. This resource was developed to be used as a central store for all policies and guidelines relating to medical needs, similar to the child protection folder that schools have. The information is regularly reviewed and updated.
- development of local guidelines in line with national guidance. These guidelines are agreed by the local authority
- co-ordination role with services such as the ambulance service and Pharmacists.
- offer general medical needs training to all education staff working on school sites. There is an increasing number of schools with extended provisions eg. breakfast clubs and after-school clubs and staff working within these settings should also receive training
- co-ordinate and keep records of training provided to staff and the need for training to be up-dated

Nurse specialists from local acute services and community children's nurses undertake training for education staff on particular complex care procedures, eg. care of a child with a tracheostomy or a child requiring intermittent catheterisation.

**Oxfordshire** has developed shared training protocols for the care of children in any setting. The protocols have been developed and agreed by a multi-agency group representing education, social services, health and the voluntary sector. The aim was to ensure that all staff would be trained to a consistent level of competence and that the training would be to a high standard and be provided by the most appropriate professional. This approach ensures that staff are protected legally and that children receive a service which is consistent in all settings.

The model is based on categorising every care task into one of five levels of training. Care tasks cover a comprehensive range of tasks from assisting a child with eating and drinking or assisting with intimate care through to tracheostomy and stoma care.

- Level 1 and 2: For these care tasks the care worker will have received general, basic training from their employer and/or health care professional. These are transferable skills. Level 2 tasks are classified to meet a health need. Level 1 includes tasks such as the disposal of clinical waste and intimate care. Examples of Level 2 tasks are moving and handling and care during menstruation.

- Level 3 and 4: These are health care tasks and require a specific care worker to receive training for a 'named' child. The training is provided by a health care professional. The trainee must be assessed as competent to undertake the task and documentation be signed by the health professional to indicate this. At the time of assessment of competence monitoring and training update will be agreed. Level 4 tasks are perceived as complex and complicated health care tasks. Examples of Level 3 tasks include the administration of medication via a nebuliser and wet wrapping for a child with eczema. Level 4 tasks include the care of children on oxygen and stoma care.
- For Level 3 and 4 tasks service level agreements will be arranged between appropriate services
- Level 5: These tasks can only be carried out by a health care professional; a care worker cannot undertake them. Parents must be offered training by a health care professional so that they can feel confident, competent and adequately supported so that they can care for their child at home. Tasks at this level include dialysis and the replacement of a gastrostomy tube.

The training responsibilities of health care professionals and the way in which verification of training and competency is assessed will then vary according to the level at which a task has been categorised. For example:

**example**

- Level 2: Training may be given by either the employing agency or by a health care professional, dependant on the task or policy. Monitoring of the care worker is the responsibility of the employing agency.
- Level 3 and 4: The health care professional's role is to advise, train and agree competence. The health care professional provides written guidelines and monitors of the care worker for the agreed specific care task.

The training protocols tend to follow the same format throughout. Examples of protocols for care tasks at Level 2 (changing of incontinence pads and nappies) and Level 4 (Bolus naso-gastric feeding) are given at the end of this chapter to illustrate the system used by Oxfordshire.

### Moving and handling

As highlighted in chapter 5 on risk assessment, staff supporting children who require moving and handling will require specific training. As with other areas of training, general information and specific training in relation to an individual's needs will be required.

No-one should carry out any moving and handling procedure until they have received accredited training and been deemed competent. Training should always be provided by an accredited trainer and cannot be cascaded. It is important that trainers have experience in the specific needs of children. Employers need to offer regular opportunities for staff to update their training. Training should cover both safe and unsafe lifting.

Where equipment is available in schools and early years settings to assist with moving and handling, it is important the staff receive training on using pieces of equipment for specific children. Equipment, such as hoists and overhead tracking must be regularly serviced and maintained. There should be an agreement as to who owns the equipment as well as who is responsible for maintaining and servicing it.

Following the training of staff in moving and handling for a specific child, those instructions on each move should be clearly written down. An example of this is contained in the completed risk assessment on manual handling at the end of chapter 5.

### Competence

Once a staff member has been trained, the health professional conducting the training should sign to state that the person is competent to carry out a particular procedure and agree when the training should be updated. The 'Staff training record – administration of medicines', taken from the *Managing medicines in schools and early years settings* guidance can be used for this purpose. A copy of that form is to be found at the end of this chapter.

An example of good practice is a method of training which has been developed based on a competency model of learning and assessment in order to overcome some of the difficulties which health staff perceive when agreeing competence. The model has been developed to be used to train non-health staff in the areas covered by the North Warwickshire PCT, South Warwickshire PCT, Coventry PCT and Rugby PCT. The following describes the approach taken:

**example** *This approach is based on Steinaker and Bells model of learning (1979).[1] It acknowledges the different phases of learning. It is comprehensive and can be used to train and assess parents, carers, classroom assistants, less experienced nurses and the nurses teaching the skill.*

*It is child orientated and encourages the teaching of a holistic set of skills. Using a psychological approach, gaining age appropriate consent and recognising the child's privacy are all important elements in this model. The documents used in this method have been reviewed by the legal advisors of the health care trust. This has given confidence to those being trained and trust staff that they are safe to use them. This approach has led to the same documents being used throughout the child's life, in various settings, the hospital, home, school, short break care, and foster care giving a high level of consistency.*

1 N. W. Steinaker and M. R. Bell (1979). *The experiential taxonomy: a new approach to teaching and learning.* New York: Academic Press

The training and assessment for each procedure taught is based on a number of competencies and individuals being trained and assessed can achieve competence on a number of different levels. These levels are:
- initial training
- practical training
- competent to practice
- competent and experienced
- competent to teach

A summary of the training material and competency assessment used to train staff is included at the end of this chapter.

Included at the end of this chapter are:

7.1 Examples of two training protocols from Oxfordshire

7.2 Staff training record from Managing Medicines in Schools and Early Years settings

7.3 Training material and Competency assessments used by the health trusts in Warwickshire, Coventry and Rugby

### 2.4  Changing of incontinence pads and nappies

**Training to be given by**
- Employing agency
- Children's nurse
- Continence advisory service

**Criteria for training**
The care worker must have received Level 1 training in Guidelines for intimate and Personal care in the community setting and Level 2 Moving and handling training prior to undertaking the task.

**Specific issues to be covered in training**
- Privacy and dignity
- How to change a nappy for an infant, and a pad for the older child with continence problems
- The importance of promoting independence and continence
- Continence products available
- Disposal of continence products

**Written information and documentation which needs to be in place**
To cover the above

**Method of assessment**
To be decided by the employing agency

**Monitoring**
At the discretion of the employing agency – every two years is suggested

### Guidelines for training

*Procedure*
1. Explain what you are going to do to the child/young person
2. Establish whether the child/young person lies down or stands up
3. Take/guide the child/young person to the bedroom/bathroom
4. Ensure dignity and privacy are respected
5. The wearing of disposable gloves is recommended
6. Only lower essential garments
7. Remove pad/nappy and dispose of appropriately
8. When washing/wiping always do this from front to back to prevent any infection
9. Ensure skin is dry
10. Replace fresh pad/nappy
11. Encourage child/young person to wash their hand
12. Tidy changing area
13. Wash own hands

### 4.3 Bolus naso-gastric feeding

## Training to be given by
- Children's nurse

## Criteria for training
- Child must be able to tolerate feeds well
- To be assessed by nurse prior to training being agreed
- If medication is to be given, then the care worker must have received Level 3 training 'Administration of medications' relevant to employing agency
- Passing of a tube and continuous/overnight feeding are Level 5 tasks
- A risk assessment re complexity of confirming correct positioning of tube must have been completed

## Specific issues to be covered in training
- Basic and relevant anatomy and physiology
- Possible problems of naso-gastric feeding and how to manage these
- How to secure the tube to the child's face
- How to test correct positioning of tube and action to take if unable to confirm correct positioning
- Equipment to be used
- Feed being used
- How to give feed
- Action to take if child coughs or vomits during feed
- Hygiene

## Written information and documentation which needs to be in place
- Written information should include all the above points and be individualised for each child
- Included in the care plan should be contact number of nurse

## Method of assessment
The naso-gastric feed should be demonstrated at least once and the care worker be observed a minimum of once before being assessed as competent

## Monitoring
Monitoring and reassessment should be undertaken on a six monthly basis or if the child's requirements change

### Guidelines for training

A naso-gastric tube is a tube, made of plastic or silk, which is passed through a nostril, down the oesophagus into the stomach. It is used as a short term measure when a baby or child is unable to take any or sufficient nutrition orally. The tube is secured to the child's face with tape.

### Equipment

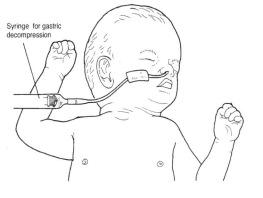

Syringe for gastric decompression

- 50ml luer lock syringe
- Strip of testing paper
- 10ml syringe filled with water
- Feed

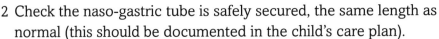

*Procedure*

1 Prior to commencing feed ensure the child is comfortable and in their preferred position.
2 Check the naso-gastric tube is safely secured, the same length as normal (this should be documented in the child's care plan).
3 Wash hands.
4 Take off port cover at end of naso-gastric tube. Attach 50ml syringe, with 3-10mls air in it. Gently push air into stomach (this will encourage the tube to move away from the lining of the stomach). Gently pull back plunger and aspirate a small amount of stomach contents. If unable to obtain aspirate, change child's position and retry. If still unsuccessful and child is allowed to drink then offer them some fluids, wait 10 minutes and try again. If unable to obtain any aspirate then contact parent/relevant professional – DO NOT CONTINUE WITH FEED.
5 Once some aspirate has been obtained, disconnect syringe from naso-gastric tube and replace port cover.
6 Squirt aspirate onto testing paper and check if the colour changes as advised.
7 Remove plunger from 50ml syringe. Reconnect syringe to naso-gastric tube. Kink tube to prevent air entering stomach.
8 Fill syringe with feed, unkink tube and use gravity to allow feed to run in.
9 As the syringe begins to empty, fill up with more feed – so that the syringe is never empty until the end of the feed.
10 Feeding should take 15–20 minutes.
11 If feed will not run, try elevating syringe to increase gravity, or try pushing on plunger to start feed and then disconnect. Check tube is not kinked.
12 When feed is finished, disconnect 50ml syringe and connect 10ml syringe. Flush tube with water. Disconnect and replace port cover.

13 Wash syringes in warm soapy water, rinse and leave to air dry. If child is under one or has been advised by a health care professional to do so, sterilise according to instructions and then store dry until needed. Reusable syringes may be used up to 30 times.

## Trouble shooting

- If the child feels sick, or has a fit or is unwell, stop feeding for a short while and, if possible, restart later.
- If the tube is dislodged during the feed discontinue immediately and inform parents.

# Staff training record from 'Managing medicines in schools and early years settings'

Name of school/setting ——————————————————————————

Name ——————————————————————————————————

Type of training received ——————————————————————————

Date of training completed ——————————————————————————

Training provided by ————————————————————————————

Profession and title —————————————————————————————

I confirm that [name of member of staff] has received the training detailed above and is competent to carry out any necessary treatment. I recommend that the training is updated [please state how often].

Trainer's signature ————————————————————————————

Date ———————————————————————————————————

**I confirm that I have received the training detailed above.**

Staff signature —————————————————————————————————

Date ———————————————————————————————————

Suggested review date ————————————————————————————

# Training material and competency assessments used by the health trusts in Warwickshire, Coventry and Rugby

This competency is for _____ only.

## This competency expires on _____

This competency certifies carer _____ only.

## Areas of concern

- Basic anatomy and physiology
- Psychological implications
- Demonstration of skill
- Complications and trouble shooting
- Safety routines
- Record keeping (DoH 2001b)
- Privacy and dignity (DoH 2001b)

## Required skills and knowledge

Each area of concern is broken down into its own component parts, grouped into sections and signed by worker and teacher/assessor when completed at each of the following levels.

## Levels of competency

- Exposure – initial teaching
- Participation – supervised practice
- Identification – safe to practice
- Internalisation – competent/confident practice (risk of over confidence)
- Dissemination – safe to teacher/research (Steinaker & Bell 1979).

Individual levels assessed by

Name _____ Initial _____

Signature _____

**I certify that the person named, as carer on this document is competent to carry out the procedure detailed above and that I have current NMC registration.**

Overall competency _____

Date _____

I the above named carer certify that I am happy to carry out the above procedure within the competencies detailed above. I understand the scope of these competencies. I will only use this training in respect of the child specifically named on the front of this form and I will not carry out procedures, which are contrary to or not covered by this training.

I will seek further training if I have any concerns about my competency and in any event six weeks before the expiry date on the front of this form renew my training. Upon the date of expiry of this competency, if my training has not been renewed, or if I have concerns about my competency, I will discontinue undertaking the procedure detailed in this document and seek appropriate advice from a suitably qualified clinician and or my employer. In all other respects I will seek all necessary advice guidance and further training needed from time to time in order for me to continue to operate within these competencies.

Name _____

Signature _____

Date _____

**Employers of non-NHS trainees**

We will use our best endeavours to ensure that our employee/staff member delivers care to the person named within the boundaries of this competency as outlined above.

Name _____

Designation _____

Signature _____

Date _____

# 8 Support arrangements

A number of children with complex health need will require one to one support whilst at school or in an early years setting. The level of support required by a child should be clearly stated in both the statement of special educational needs (where there is one) and in the individual health care plan.

The funding for this support is likely to come from either health or education or may be jointly funded. One of the issues likely to arise is that of joint governance where health staff are employed in an education setting.

This chapter details a number of examples of flexible support arrangements in different settings.

The first case study describes the work in the Phoenix Pre-School Centre in Bromley, illustrating flexible and creative use of the support role.

**example**

*The Phoenix Children's Resource Centre in **Bromley**, hosts services working with young children with special needs and disabilities. The centre is remodelling the workforce to pioneer and develop new integrated care pathways. New dual worker roles enable young disabled children with complex health needs to receive both medical/care support and full access to the Foundation Stage Curriculum. The new roles have developed from the work of the Bromley Early Support Programme. This places the child and family at the centre of co-ordinated service delivery, and provides support at the Phoenix Centre, in the family's home and in mainstream inclusive pre-school settings across the Borough.*

*Edward is a three year-old attending class-based provision at the Phoenix Children's Resource Centre. He has been receiving co-ordinated support from 13 different services through the Bromley Early Support Programme. This includes an early support keyworker. Edward and his family require help to meet his complex medical care needs, which include severe epilepsy and the need for gastrostomy tube feeding. He also requires extra help to achieve full access to the Foundation Stage Curriculum. As an extension of the Early Support Programme and in order to provide a co-ordinated family friendly response to joint assessment, the Phoenix Centre is pioneering a new dual worker role, whereby staff are trained to work with young disabled children and their families and meet both their medical/health care and Foundation Stage educational needs.*

*Edward now has a trained dual worker who can go to his home in the* morning and support the family with his gastrostomy feed, personal care and getting him ready to go to the Phoenix Pre-School Centre classrooms. Whilst at the Centre, the dual worker supports Edward's access to the Foundation Stage Curriculum, suitably modified to meet his needs. Extra support and access for communication includes use of touch cues and switches and physical prompts. Other specialist equipment provides physical access to all areas including the Sensory Room. For positioning and posture, Edward requires a special spinal jacket, a standing frame, a Saturn chair, a lying board and wedge for chest percussion as well as therapy support. The dual worker also importantly ensures that his medical/care needs are met, which for Edward includes gastrostomy tube feeding, setting up the pump, checking his tummy for air, flushing the gastrostomy peg with water and administering the tube feed. These medical processes are outlined in Edward's health care plan, which includes a plan for epilepsy management and oral care. Training and supervision for Edward's dual worker was provided by a specialist nurse trainer and once the dual worker was assessed as both confident and competent in procedures, the protocols were 'signed off' by both the parents and nurse trainer. The dual worker works as part of the team in the class and not exclusively with Edward.

The multi-agency team working at the Phoenix Centre has looked beyond traditional work boundaries and has rethought access to services and support for both Edward and his family. For example, a teaching assistant would have traditionally waited for Edward to arrive at the Phoenix Pre-School classrooms in the morning. The dual worker can go home and support the family in getting him ready and into school. The development and piloting of new roles and systems to support medical/care needs as well as educational needs has meant the Phoenix multi-agency team have needed to address issues such as:

- establishing joint job descriptions and evaluations
- pay and conditions
- new recruitment protocols
- training competencies being signed off and agreed by Bromley PCT, LEA and the parents
- joint risk assessments
- joint funding and monitoring protocols
- multi-agency single access referral pathways
- health care plans and new information to parents
- consideration of indemnification issues

Edward and his family have been placed at the centre of service delivery. This has included earlier involvement of the family as the new processes have been piloted and Family Service Plans and health care plans were developed.

Other features of the scheme include a new multi-agency Internet accessible database and means of data collection, extended specialist roles for nurses as trainers, joint consideration of core skills for dual workers with knowledge and competencies including moving and handling training, use of and access to equipment both at home and at the Centre and managing technological equipment. The team have been supported by a cross-agency management commitment to new ways of working as part of the 'Every Child Matters' agenda.

The multi-agency team is working with Edward and his family to assess his overall needs, both medical and educational, before consideration of any statutory assessment processes which will take place just prior to Edward moving from the Phoenix and starting school at rising five.

The dual worker pilot has been so successful that the multi-agency team is now looking at rolling out the procedures to inclusive mainstream pre-school settings, which in Bromley are mostly in the private and voluntary sector, to ensure all training and processes are in place to support medical needs before the child starts school.

The second case study describes a child accessing mainstream education in Kingston upon Thames who requires two support staff to assist on a full time basis:

**example** Sam is six years old and has a diagnosis of hereditary motor and sensor neuropathy type 2. He has very little independent movement other than head turning. He has a **tracheostomy** and a **gastrostomy** and is **ventilated 24 hours a day**. His prognosis is unknown although it was not originally expected that Sam would achieve school age.

In spite of his considerable physical needs Sam is well motivated to learn and communicate. He is making good progress in school and is achieving at above average levels in comparison to his mainstream peers.

Sam was first referred to the local education authority at the age of one when the **Portage** service became involved. At that time he was supported at home by the **home ventilation team**. His care was co-ordinated by a member of this team who oversaw the budget which the Hospital Trust had set aside for this purpose. He was referred to the local education authority as a child who would require specialist provision to access school.

When Sam was three years old the statutory assessment process began, involving health, education and social services. Sam's parents were clear that although the local education authority had a special school for children with physical disabilities, their preference was for Sam to attend his local nursery and then mainstream infant school. The school visited Sam and his family at home and made a commitment to supporting him in a mainstream placement. His placement would be jointly funded by health and education.

Sam needed two support workers, both employed by the hospital trust on health pay scales, but one funded by this Trust and the other by the local education authority. They would both be managed on a day-to-day basis by the head teacher. Both workers would be trained to suction, hand ventilate, use a hoist, etc. Appropriate training would be provided by both health and education. A pooled budget was set up. The education authority purchased the necessary ICT and communication system. Risk assessments were carried out. Building work was undertaken well in advance; first the nursery and then the classroom and toilet area in the reception building were adapted.

The process has been a learning experience for all the agencies involved. The main challenges have been the increasing difficulties with the deployment of health staff to support Sam in school. Sam requires minimal cognitive support. His needs are around his physical access to the curriculum in terms of presentation of task, recording ,etc. health staff have been resistant to work in this area, despite training. The local education authority have tried various arrangements, some of which have led to an in-equality of work load. At the time of writing this case study It is proposed that both posts may in future be recruited and employed by Sam's junior school but with health retaining the funding one of the posts and providing training for both posts.

Many of the decisions have been pragmatic solutions to the challenges and difficulties which have arisen. However, supporting Sam to access mainstream education has shown a commitment to achieving inclusion by the family and agencies involved.

The third example focuses on the work of the inclusion support service in Enfield.

**example** This service has a varied role which includes the provision of education and continuity for sick children, be they in hospital, at home or in school. In addition it has a team of support assistants and teachers including those working with sensory impairment that can be deployed to assist pupils, parents and schools with the inclusion of a child who needs considerable support or unusual support. These staff are experienced and well trained to work with children who have complex health needs.

The staff may simply provide emergency cover to ensure a child is in school with the necessary support and care until the school personnel have the necessary training and confidence to take over. The Service can facilitate the development of a care plan and will liaise closely with the health trust to organize training for insulin injections, rectal diazepam administration, etc.

A member of staff from the central team works with the child while the school is encouraged to take over the responsibility when it is ready and this allow the support assistant to move on. However the situation may not always be resolved quickly.

Recently a school was requested to admit a reception child with an unstable diabetes that was being treated with very frequent injections and blood tests. The school and parents had concerns about the situation. The central team provided a support assistant, who had additional training. After a year of support from the central team and work liasing between parents, health providers, the school and local authority staff the school will now take over the care of the child with its own trained staff.

Enfield's experience has shown that it is sometimes difficult for schools to appoint staff who can be both learning support assistants and provide of high dependency care to pupils. Intimate care such as catheterisation, toileting, physiotherapy routines are not always within the normal skills of a teaching assistant. It is for this reason that Enfield keeps a core team of special support assistants who can be deployed where needed.

They not only support the pupil but can help the school develop practices towards SEN pupils. They are often the link with parents and can facilitate progression to further and higher education. In cases where the condition is deteriorating they may become very important to the parent and child.

Work of this sort places considerable demands on staff and it is for this reason that they have opportunities to be supported by their manager and meet with other members of the team.

The fourth example illustrates the need for many children, particularly older children, to receive support in a way that is sensitive to a child's growing independence and their need to interact with their peers. There needs to be a balance between ensuring the safety of children and allowing them to lead a valued and dignified life.

**example** In North Yorkshire, this balance was achieved for a young person in high school who was given a simple pager. This gave him the independence to interact with his peers during breaks whilst at the same time he had a quick and easy way to call his support assistant when he required help.

### Trips and outside activities

It is considered good practice to ensure that children with complex health needs are able to participate in off-site trips, visits and activities. In addition to the risk assessments which would be carried out for any off-site activity, further risk assessments may be required to assess the suitability of the activity and venue. Reasonable adjustments may need to be made to enable children with complex health needs to participate fully and safely in activities. Staff supervising an off-site visit or activity should be aware of the support children with complex health needs may require both routinely and in the case of an emergency. A copy of the health care plan should be taken on visits. In any risk assessment for off-site visits it is important not to rely on mobile phones as the only form of communication as there are parts of the countryside where mobile phone reception remains inadequate.

*Issues arising from off-site trips and visits are discussed in Exemplars 2 and 4 (Gareth and Daniel)*

A step-by-step guide used by Nottinghamshire Education Department has been included at the end of this chapter. This illustrates what schools and other settings need to do over and above their usual risk assessments.

Included at the end of this chapter is:
8.1 Checklist for off-site visits from Nottingham Education Department

### Step 1
SENCO and EVC meet annually to review all planned visits to identify pupils with SEN and known disabilities within school population, and their potential to be invited on educational visits.

### Step 2
Inform visit leaders of potential pupil needs in target groups.

### Step 3
Initial planning and risk assessment of visit.

### Step 4
Visit leader with help from SENCO and EVC consider if visit is inclusive for potential pupil group, make early consideration of need to adjust if necessary. Make anticipatory adjustments.

### Step 5
In first communications with parents invite them to contribute information of their child's additional needs/medical need/disability, which may impact on the organisation of the visit.

For residential visits invite parents to provide information which may not be apparent in the school day.

### Step 6
Using problem solving focused approach consider the needs of known pupils in relation to transport, accommodation, activities, staffing ratios, timetables, other.

### Step 7
Consider reasonableness of proposed adjustments and discuss with parents.
*or*
Consider alternative activity.

### Step 8
Review the effectiveness of reasonableness of adjustments and/or alternative arrangements once visit complete.

# 9 Other issues

This chapter deals with a number of specific issues which may arise when supporting children with complex health needs:
- catering
- continence
- facilities
- infection control
- transport
- emergency treatment
- altered states of health

## Catering

Children with complex health needs may have specific dietary requirements. These requirements may relate to:
- allergies to certain foods
- the way food is prepared and given, for example children who are tube fed.

*Exemplar 1 (Kamahl) describes issues which arise for children who are gastrostomy fed.*

The *Managing medicines in schools and early years settings* (DfES/DH, 2005) details information relating to Anaphylaxis and further information can be found at www.alllergyinschools.org.uk.

In order to provide a safe and supportive environment for children with specific needs, schools and early years settings should:
- have a policy which outlines how to provide a catering service which ensures the safe inclusion of children with specific dietary requirements
- collect the information about the needs of children with complex health needs during the admission process. An example of a form developed by an early years setting in Bolton is included at the end of this chapter.
- provide clear information for staff involved in food preparation and supporting children during meal times
- provide additional training for staff involved in food preparation and meal supervision
- ensure the safety of children, where necessary by sharing information with other children and young people.

## Continence

Most children develop continence prior to attending nursery or school. Some children with complex health needs may never achieve this. The Disability Discrimination Act (DDA) requires all education providers to re-examine all policies, consider the implications of the Act for practice, and revise their current arrangements. In the light of historical practices that no longer comply with new legislation, changes will particularly be required wherever blanket rules about continence have been a feature of a setting/school's admissions policy. It is unacceptable to refuse admission to children who are delayed in achieving continence. Schools and settings will also need to set in motion action that ensures they provide an accessible toileting facility if this has not previously been available. The Department of Health has issued clear guidance about the facilities that should be available in each school. (*Good practice in continence services*, DH, 2000).

The guidance states systems of care should be put in place that:
- *Preserve the dignity and independence of the child or young person and avoids the risk of ridicule or bullying from peers or staff*
- *Carry out the continence treatment or management plan as agreed in the assessment;*
- *Enable good pathways of communication from child or young person to the school-based carer, the multi-disciplinary team and the parent or carer*
- *Provide adequately trained school-based care staff*

Local authorities and other employers should consider developing policies and protocols which will assist schools and other settings to ensure that children are not excluded; and there are adequate facilities; and risk assessments are in place. An example of a policy developed by Leicester City Local Education Authority is included at the end of this chapter.

Incontinence may create a lot of embarrassment for children or young people, particularly as they get older. Children may be reluctant to discuss their condition and may be worried about attention being drawn to it in any way. Aspects of the day which are particularly difficult are sports activities and off-site events, particularly if they include an overnight stay. Some schools, particularly secondary schools, have developed 'smartcard' systems so that a child can show a card to a member of staff if they need to use the toilet, without having to go into a long explanation in front of their peers.

A good policy should:
- place continence in the context of disability discrimination legislation. It should give a commitment to ensuring the inclusion of this group of children in all activities
- ensure the dignity, independence, need for privacy and self esteem of the child or young person at all times

- be linked to an anti-bullying policy
- define the health and safety issues, for example the use of protective garments and the disposal of clinical waste
- outline the facilities which should be in place to ensure the privacy and dignity of the children. Facilities may need to be adapted to encourage independence and ensure privacy
- define the procedures or protocols which should be followed during personal or intimate care. These may form part of the health care plan and should be child centred, encourage the independence and address issues of confidentiality which the child or young person may request.
- highlight the child protection issues which need to be taken into account

### Facilities

As the population of children with complex health needs changes so the physical environment and facilities available in various settings will have to alter to meet the changing needs. Through accessibility planning schools should develop plans to change the physical environment to meet the needs of children with complex health needs.

*Both Exemplars 2 and 3 (Gareth and Anita) describe some of the changes which may be needed for children with complex health needs.*

The type of facilities which will need to be available are outlined in a report to the National Assembly for Wales:
- *Require areas that can be maintained as sterile*
- *Offer sufficient space for the safe storage, retrieval, servicing and deployment of equipment, wheelchairs, etc*
- *Ensure privacy for the provision of intimate care or medical treatment or therapy.*
- *Have safe storage arrangements for medication*
- *Have quiet places for children who are feeling unwell, recovering from an epileptic fit or treatment*
- *Have efficient heating, as severely disabled children are unlikely to be sufficiently mobile to keep warm and are likely to spend periods of time on the floor or in fixed equipment or wheelchairs, Cleanliness and warmth are essential to their well-being*
- *Have safe access arrangements for wheelchairs and mobility aids, transport vehicles and outside play areas.*

(Russell *et al*, 2002. p.21)

### Infection control

As part of a general health and safety policy employers should have a policy covering infection control.

*Exemplar 2 (Gareth) highlights some of the issues relating to infection control.*

Standard measures to ensure the most basic level of infection control will include:
- good hygiene practice – washing and drying hands
- use of protective barriers, for example, gloves and aprons
- safe handling of sharps
- use of sterile techniques

The local authority may assist schools and other settings by producing guidelines, for example, Lancashire Education Authority guidelines on basic hygiene practices can be found at the end of this chapter.

## Transport

Some children with complex health needs will require the local authority to provide transport to and from school. Guidance for education can be found in *Home to school travel for pupils requiring special arrangements*. (DfES, November 2004). The guidance sets out a checklist of minimum standards that should apply to all special transport services. Other settings may provide transport for off-site visits.

In line with the above guidance all schools and early years settings should:
- use transport which ensures the inclusion of children with complex health needs and children who use wheelchairs
- when assessing and managing risk, the responsible officer must take into account additional needs, which include medical/health needs.
- all drivers and escorts must have first aid training and additional training should be provided to escorts who are required to support pupils with complex health needs
- all vehicles should have a means of communication available to use in emergencies
- drivers and escorts should know what to do in the case of an emergency. Where this entails the administration of medication or other procedures they should be appropriately trained and supported. Staff transporting children who are at risk of anaphylactic shock should be trained in the use of epipens for emergencies.
- accredited training courses should be offered to all drivers and escorts. Information on accredited courses can be found on the Community Transport Association website (www.comunitytransport.com).
- where appropriate, the child's health care plan should be carried in the transport with the child.

## Emergency treatment

All schools and other settings should have first aid policies and procedures in place that cover all emergencies. Guidance on first aid in schools can be found on the DfES website: www.teachernet.gov.uk/firstaid. First aiders must complete a training course approved by the Health and Safety Executive. The number of first aiders will depend on specific circumstances and should be based on a risk assessment. The main duties of a first aider are to:

- give immediate help to casualties with common injuries or illnesses and those arising from specific hazards at school
- when necessary, ensure that an ambulance or other professional medical help is called.

For children with complex health needs, their individual health care plan should cover emergency situations. It is important that this information is carried with the child or is easily accessible and that it is written in a format that is easily understood and can be followed at a time of crisis.

Examples of two plans used at St Margaret's School in Surrey demonstrate the type of format that will be easy to follow in an emergency (included at the end of this chapter).

### Summon assistance in an emergency

There are a number of examples of creative ideas used in order for a teacher or playground staff member to summon assistance if he/she is alone in a classroom with a group of children and there is an emergency involving one child. The purpose behind these systems is to send another child to summon help carrying an easily identifiable object rather than relying on a child to carry a verbal message. The two examples given here are:

- a card alert procedure recommended by the Learning Trust in Hackney.
- the helping hand system recommended by the nurses responsible for medical needs in the South Birmingham Primary Care Trust

### The card alert procedure

A warning card is available in the classroom to alert any member of staff to the information they may need relating to a specific child. As SOS card is available in the classroom and held by lunchtime and playground staff which in the event of an emergency is given to another child to take to a designated place – usually the school office. The staff in the office will be respond by ensuring that medication and a trained person is taken to the emergency situation.

### The helping hand system

A large cardboard hand (about 20 inches in height) is kept in each classroom, with the name of the class printed on it. In the case of an emergency, another child is given the hand and sent to a designated place – usually the office. The 'hand' is obvious because of its size and the child carrying it can be easily seen and responded to.

At the time of writing one of the major issues challenging schools and local authorities is that of 'do not resuscitate orders'. A 'Do not resuscitate' order (DNR) is an agreement drawn up between a child's parents and the medical staff with clinical responsibility for the child. It authorises or denies treatment where it is agreed as being in the best interests of the child. Where a DNR order exists, this must be discussed at the meeting arranged to draw up the health care plan and clearly stated in the plan. A copy of the DNR order should be kept in a place which can be accessed in an emergency. The ambulance service should be made aware of children who have DNR orders.

In an emergency situation staff must phone for an ambulance, inform relevant health professionals who are on site and notify the parents. Making decisions relating to a child in this situation is a clinical matter and not one that can be made by staff in schools or early years settings. Whilst, staff can tell parents that they respect the DNR order, they cannot make decisions relating to the treatment of the child. School or early years staff are not responsible for any decisions made by health professionals.

## Altered states of health

A small number of children do not maintain a high level of health and well being. It is often difficult for staff to gauge whether these children are ill or their state is 'normal' for them. It is important that these children are not regularly being sent home on health grounds, but that staff work with parents and health professionals to get to know them well before making a judgement that they are ill and need to be sent home.

Included at the end of this chapter are:
9.1  Safe food agreement – Bolton early years team
9.2  Continence policy – Leicester City Local Education Authority
9.3  Infection control information – Lancashire Education Authority
9.4  Emergency protocol for seizures – St Margaret's School
9.5  Emergency protocol for pain – St Margaret's School

Child's name _____

Date of birth _____

Attendance _____

photograph

Brief account of child's intolerances

_____

_____

_____

We give staff at _____ permission to give _____
the following foods

Meat _____

Vegetables _____

Fruit _____

Others _____

This list will be updated when advised of new safe foods which have been tried at home for a minimum of five times with no side effects.

*Signed*

Parent _____ Parent _____

Date _____

We agree to do all we can to ensure that only the above foods
are offered to _____

*Signed*

Manager _____ Room leader _____

Cook _____ Cook _____

Nursery nurse _____

**NB  To be kept where food is prepared and consumed**

The Disability Discrimination Act (DDA) requires all education providers to re-examine all policies, consider the implications of the Act for practice and revise their current arrangements. In the light of historical practices that no longer comply with new legislation, changes will particularly be required wherever blanket rules about continence have been a feature of a setting/school's admissions policy. Schools and settings will also need to set in motion action that ensures they provide an accessible toileting facility if this has not previously been available. The Department of Health has issued clear guidance about the facilities that should be available in each school (Good Practice in Continence Services, 2000).

Achieving continence is one of hundreds of developmental milestones usually reached within the context of learning in the home before the child transfers to learning in a nursery/school setting. In some cases this one developmental area has assumed significance beyond all others. Parents are sometimes made to feel guilty that this aspect of learning has not been achieved, whereas other delayed learning is not so stigmatising.

## Definition of disability in DDA

The DDA provides protection for anyone who has a physical, sensory or mental impairment that has an adverse effect on his/her ability to carry out normal day-to-day activities. The effect must be substantial and long-term.

It is clear therefore that anyone with a named condition that affects aspects of personal development must not be discriminated against. However, it is also unacceptable to refuse admission to other children who are delayed in achieving continence. Delayed continence is not necessarily linked with learning difficulties. However, children with global developmental delay which may not have been identified by the time they enter nursery or school are likely to be late coming out of nappies.

Education providers have an obligation to meet the needs of children with delayed personal development in the same way as they would meet the individual needs of children with delayed language, or any other kind of delayed development. Children should not be excluded from normal pre-school activities solely because of incontinence.

Any admission policy that sets a blanket standard of continence, or any other aspect of development, for all children is discriminatory and therefore unlawful under the Act. All such issues have to be dealt with on an individual basis, and settings/schools are expected to make reasonable adjustments to meet the needs of each child.

*Schools and settings should consider the following issues:*

### Health and safety

Schools and all other settings registered to provide education will already have Hygiene or Infection Control policies as part of their Health and Safety policy. This is a necessary statement of the procedures the setting/school will follow in case a child accidentally wets or soils him/herself, or is sick while on the premises. The same precautions will apply for nappy changing.

This is likely to include:
- staff to wear disposable gloves and aprons while dealing with the incident
- soiled nappies to be double wrapped, or placed in a hygienic disposal unit if the number produced each week exceeds that allowed by Health and Safety Executive's limit
- changing area to be cleaned after use
- hot water and liquid soap available to wash hands as soon as the task is completed
- hot air dryer or paper towels available for drying hands

Asking parents of a child to come and change a child is likely to be a direct contravention of the DDA, and leaving a child in a soiled nappy for any length of time pending the return of the parent is a form of abuse.

### Facilities

Playgroups and schools are now admitting younger children, some of whom who, by virtue of their immaturity, are likely to have occasional accidents, especially in the first few months after admission. Current DfES recommendations for purpose built foundation stage units include an area for changing and showering children in order to meet the personal development needs of young children. There is also evidence that there is a trend for the parents of children with more complex needs to request a place for their child in a mainstream school. A suitable place for changing children therefore, should have a high priority in any setting's/school's Access Plan. The Department of Health recommends that one extended cubicle with a wash basin should be provided in each school for children with disabilities. If it is not possible to provide a purpose built changing area, then it is possible to purchase a changing mat, and change the child on the floor or on another suitable surface. A 'Do not enter' sign (visually illustrated) can be placed on the toilet door to ensure that privacy and dignity are maintained during the time taken to change the child. Clean, fresh water drinking facilities should be available at all times.

### Child protection

The normal process of changing a nappy should not raise child protection concerns, and there are no regulations that indicate that a

*Including me*

second member of staff must be available to supervise the nappy changing process to ensure that abuse does not take place. Few setting/schools will have the staffing resources to provide two members of staff for nappy changing and CRB checks are carried out to ensure the safety of children with staff employed in childcare and education settings. If there is known risk of false allegation by a child then a single practitioner should not undertake nappy changing. A student on placement should not change a nappy unsupervised.

Setting/school managers are encouraged to remain highly vigilant for any signs or symptom of improper practice, as they do for all activities carried out on site.

### Agreeing a procedure for personal care in your setting/school

Settings/schools should have clear written guidelines for staff to follow when changing a child, to ensure that staff follow correct procedures and are not worried about false accusations of abuse. Parents should be aware of the procedures the school will follow should their child need changing during school time.

Your written guidelines will specify:
• who will change the nappy
• where nappy changing will take place
• what resources will be used (cleansing agents used or cream to be applied?)
• how the nappy will be disposed of
• what infection control measures are in place
• what the staff member will do if the child is unduly distressed by the experience or if the staff member notices marks or injuries

Schools may also need to consider the possibility of special circumstances arising, should a child with complex continence needs be admitted. In such circumstances the child's medical practitioners will need to be closely involved in forward planning.

### Resources

Depending on the accessibility and convenience of a setting/school's facilities, it could take ten minutes or more to change an individual child. This is not dissimilar to the amount of time that might be allocated to work with a child on an individual learning target, and of course, the time spent changing the child can be a positive, learning time.

However, if several children wearing nappies enter foundation stage provision of a setting/school there could be clear resource implications. Within a school, the foundation stage teacher or co-ordinator should speak to the SENCO to ensure that additional resources from the school's delegated SEN budget are allocated to the foundation stage group to ensure that the children's individual needs are met. With the enhanced staffing levels of provision within the private, voluntary or independent sector, allocating staff to change the children should not be such an issue, although there may be circumstances within an individual setting that merit an application for additional funding being made through the Early Years Support Link Teacher.

## Job descriptions

It is likely that most of the personal care will be undertaken by one of the teaching assistants on staff. There are some schools where teachers also take a turn with this task, but we recognise that this does not often happen. Occasionally a setting/school will say that offering personal care is not in the job descriptions of their teaching assistants. It is hard to believe how this could be the case for any assistant working with young children, and we would recommend that this be included at the next review. Certainly any new posts should have offering personal care to promote independent toileting and other self-care skills as one of the tasks.

## Keys to success

It is not helpful to assume that the child has failed to achieve full continence because the parent hasn't bothered to try. There are very few parents for whom this would be true. In the unlikely event this is the only reason why the child has not become continent then continence achievement should be uncomplicated if a positive and structured approach is used.

Remember that delayed continence may be linked with delays in other aspects of the child's development, and will benefit from a planned programme worked out in partnership with the child's parents.

There are other professionals who can help with advice and support. The School Nurse or Family Health Visitors have expertise in this area and can support parents to implement toilet training programmes in the home. Health care professionals can also carry out a full health assessment in order to rule out any medical cause of continence problems. The Specialist Community Child Health Services has produced a helpful publication 'Toileting Issues for Schools and Nurseries' which you may send for (See Further Information and Guidance) to get additional information on continence issues.

Parents are more likely to be open about their concerns about their child's learning and development and seek help, if they are confident that they and their child are not going to be judged for the child's delayed learning.

**Partnership working**

In some circumstances it may be appropriate for the setting/school to set up a home-setting/school agreement that defines the responsibilities that each partner has, and the expectations each has for the other. This might include:

- the parent
  - agreeing to ensure that the child is changed at the latest possible time before being brought to the setting/school
  - providing the setting/school with spare nappies and a change of clothing
  - understanding and agreeing the procedures that will be followed when their child is changed at school –including the use of any cleanser or the application of any cream
  - agreeing to inform the setting/school should the child have any marks/rash
  - agreeing to a 'minimum change' policy i.e. the setting/school would not undertake to change the child more frequently than if s/he were at home.
  - agreeing to review arrangements should this be necessary
- the school
  - agreeing to change the child during a single session should the child soil themselves or become uncomfortably wet
  - agreeing how often the child would be changed should the child be staying for the full day
  - agreeing to report should the child be distressed, or if marks/rashes are seen
  - agreeing to review arrangements should this be necessary.

This kind of agreement should help to avoid misunderstandings that might otherwise arise, and help parents feel confident that the setting/school is taking a holistic view of the child's needs.

### Further information and guidance

*Toileting issues for schools and nurseries* (Leicester, Leicestershire and Rutland Specialist Community Child Health Services). Available from Early Years Co-ordinator (SEN), Early Years Support Team, New Parks House, Pindar Road, Leicester LE3 9RN or e-mail early.yearssupport@leicester.gov.uk

*Enureris Resource & Information Centre* (ERIC) 34 Old School House, Britannia Road, Kingswood, Bristol BS15 8BD. Telephone 0117 960 3060, www.eric.org.uk

*Good practice in continence services*, 2000. Available free from Department of Health, PO Box 777, London SE1 6XH or www.doh.gov.uk/continenceservices.htm

## 1 Introduction

Young children in particular are prone to catching various infections throughout their early school life. There are many potential sources of infection within the home and school settings and the chief sources are likely to be as follows:

- other children or adults
- domestic and farm animals
- contaminated or uncooked food
- contaminated water

Infections can be transmitted in a variety of ways—by touch, by consuming contaminated food or water, by airborne transmission—but the main transfer of potentially unpleasant and hazardous infections within a school can be simply and effectively controlled by the establishment of good hygiene procedures. A number of strategies are likely to be involved in this respect including advice on cleaning, heating, and the use of disinfectants, but the single most effective weapon of all against the unwanted transfer of infection is hand washing.

## 2 Hand washing

Handwashing is a simple procedure which, if carried out correctly, contributes more than any other single thing to the control of infection. However, it is often neglected or carried out ineffectively. Hands should be wet thoroughly with water before applying soap. All surfaces of both hands should then be vigorously massaged with the lather.

- remember to pay special attention to the finger tips, thumbs and between the fingers as these areas are frequently missed
- right handed people have a tendency to wash the left hand more thoroughly (and vice versa). If a wedding ring is worn it is important to wash underneath it
- make sure all the soap is rinsed off under running water and then dry hands thoroughly
- always cover any cuts with a waterproof plaster
- wherever possible apply handcream as this protects hands and helps prevent dryness and chapping

Further advice and guidance on handwashing is provided on the next two pages.

Handwashing is the most important single method of controlling infection.

The hands normally have a 'resident' population of micro-organisms. Other organisms (germs) are picked up during every-day activities, and these are termed 'transient' organisms.

Many infection control problems are caused by these transient organisms.

Hand washing should remove these transient organisms before they are transferred to another pupil or to a susceptible area on the same pupil.

The potential chain of infection is broken by effective hand hygiene.

**Good practice**
- fingernails should be kept clean and short.
- ideally jewellery should not be worn
- breaks anywhere on the skin should be covered with a waterproof dressing
- medical advice should be sought for skin damage by other agents, eg eczema

**Hands should be washed**
- after visiting the toilet
- before handling food
- when hands are visibly soiled
- before a clean procedure
- after a dirty procedure, even if gloves are worn
- between care episodes for an individual pupil
- between different pupils

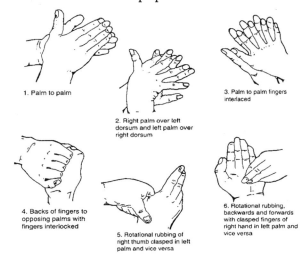

1. Palm to palm

2. Right palm over left dorsum and left palm over right dorsum

3. Palm to palm fingers interlaced

4. Backs of fingers to opposing palms with fingers interlocked

5. Rotational rubbing of right thumb clasped in left palm and vice versa

6. Rotational rubbing, backwards and forwards with clasped fingers of right hand in left palm and vice versa

### 3 Guidelines for the management of pupils with MRSA

These guidelines have been produced with the aim of providing general advice to schools on the management of pupils who are colonised with MRSA. The most effective weapons in preventing the spread of MRSA are attention to good hygiene procedures and effective handwashing techniques. It is expected that schools will already have effective hygiene procedures in place.

Where a pupil known to have MRSA is to be admitted to a **mainstream school** contact must be made with the local Community Infection Control

Nurse/Public Health Department for any necessary advice and guidance to be provided.

However, where a pupil with MRSA is to be admitted to a **special school** where he/she is likely to mix with more vulnerable pupils it is essential that a meeting should be arranged by the school involving the school nurse, the local Community Infection Control Nurse/Public Health Department representative, other appropriate representatives from the Health Services (eg health visitor, consultant community paediatrician), a representative from the LEA (if the school considers it appropriate) and the pupil's parents in order to consider any specific arrangements which may be required for the individual pupil concerned.

### 4  What is MRSA?

The initials MRSA stand for Methicillin Resistant Staphylococcus Aureus. Staphylococcus Aureus is a common bacteria and at any one time approximately one third of the population, adults and children, is colonised with them. This means that the organism lives harmlessly on a person's skin or in the nose and normally does not cause any infection beyond occasional mild skin irritations or boils. These infections are easily treated by antibiotics.

However, some strains of the Staphylococcus Aureus bacteria are resistant to the more common antibiotics and these strains are referred to under the general heading of MRSA

### 5  Who is at risk from MRSA?

MRSA can only be detected by laboratory tests and as it normally does not cause any symptoms most people will never know if they are colonised with MRSA.

MRSA may cause problems if it infects persons with surgical wounds, catheters or drips which allow bacteria to enter the body. Caution also needs to be exercised in instances where a pupil with MRSA may come into close contact with pupils who have a severely reduced resistance to infection, for instance pupils who are immuno-suppressed (e.g. pupils receiving treatment for cancer), or who have an immuno-deficient condition e.g. HIV. Further advice should be sought from the local Community Infection Control Nurse/Public Health Department in such circumstances. However, it is always worth bearing in mind that although MRSA is nowadays found not only in hospitals but also in nursing and residential homes and in the community at large, it usually only causes problems to vulnerable patients in the hospital setting.

*Including me*

## 6 Can MRSA infections be treated?

A limited number of antibiotics are still effective against MRSA infections but they can cause quite severe side effects. That is why in the UK the focus of intervention with MRSA tends to be on prevention and control. The majority of individuals with MRSA will be colonised rather than infected and so antibiotic treatment would not be necessary in any case.

## 7 Prevention and control

As with most infections, MRSA is mainly transferred by touch and so attention to good hygiene procedures and to effective handwashing techniques remain the most effective ways in which to prevent MRSA from spreading. All staff and pupils in school should be encouraged to wash their hands:

- after using the toilet
- before preparing/eating food
- after handling any soiled linen, nappies, or dressings
- after touching animals
- when hands appear or feel dirty

No special cleaning methods are required and ordinary soap is just as effective as anti-bacterial brands provided that hands are washed and dried thoroughly.

If basic good hygiene precautions are followed pupils with MRSA are not a risk to other pupils, members of staff, visitors or to members of their own families, including babies and pregnant women. Good hygiene procedures in a school setting are important to prevent the spread of all potentially infective bacteria, not just MRSA. Cutlery, toys, teaching and play materials, toilet areas and changing beds do not need to be subject to any additional hygiene precautions or procedures beyond the school's usual cleaning régime because they have been used by pupils known to be colonised with MRSA.

## 8 Points of guidance for school staff

- cuts, sores and surgical wounds in staff and pupils should be covered by a waterproof dressing to prevent infection.
- if blood or other body fluids have to be cleared up a disposable apron and disposable gloves should be worn and paper towels used. All of these items should subsequently be placed in plastic bags and disposed of safely and hygienically.
- staff who have eczema or psoriasis should not perform any intimate care procedures on pupils with MRSA.

- pupils with MRSA do not need to be taught separately from other pupils or kept in any form of isolation within the school setting.
- pupils with MRSA should be allowed to participate in out-of-school activities and visits, again with good hygiene procedures being undertaken when necessary.

## 9 Staff training

All staff who are likely to have contact with a pupil with MRSA must receive appropriate guidance on good hygiene procedures. This guidance will:
- be provided through arrangements made with the local Community Infection Control Nurse/Public Health Department (see Section 11)
- meet any specific needs of an individual pupil which are identified in collaboration with the parents, the LEA and the health professionals concerned
- be recorded on the pupil's file
- be updated on an agreed regular basis
- be recorded on the staff files

## 10 Emergency procedures

If a pupil with MRSA is to be admitted to hospital as an emergency from school (eg as a result of an accident) the ambulance personnel need to be made aware that the pupil has MRSA.

## 11 Community infection control nurses/public health departments

Each primary care trust in Lancashire should have a public health department and most trusts will employ a community infection control nurse. Colleagues in these services are in a position to offer expert advice and training to schools on any infection control problems posed by individual pupils, including those with MRSA.

It may be helpful for schools to find out in advance who the appropriate contact person would be within the local primary care trust who can advise on infection control issues.

Contact telephone numbers are as follows:
Morecambe Bay PCT    (01524) 583769
Wyre PCT    (01253) 306328
Fylde PCT    (01253) 306328
Preston PCT    (01772) 647100
Chorley & South Ribble PCT    (01772) 644479
West Lancashire PCT    (01695) 598135
Hyndburn & Ribble Valley PCT    (01254) 356800
Burnley, Pendle & Rossendale PCT    (01254) 356800

**Continuous generalised seizure**
(ie no periods of recovering
awareness for **5 mins**)
**Midazolam 2.5mg buccal**

**Marching and clusters of short
seizures** (ie recovers awareness in
between). Make comfortable, try
**paracetamol**. If lasts for **30 mins**
**Midazolam 2.5mg buccal**

If still having **continuous** seizure
activity **10 mins** after first dose
of Midazolam give
**Midazolam 2.5mg buccal**

If still having **intermittent** seizure
activity **30 mins** after first dose of
Midazolam
**Midazolam 2.5mg buccal**

If still having **continuous** seizure
activity **10 mins** after second
dose of Midazolam
**Paraldehyde 5ml PR (in 5ml oil)**

If still having **intermittent** seizure
activity **30 mins** after second dose of
Midazolam
**Paraldehyde 5ml PR (in 5ml oil)**

If still having **continuous** seizure
activity **10 mins** after Paraldehyde
**dial 999 – hospital**

If still having **intermittent** seizure
activity **30 mins** after Paraldehyde
**dial 999 – hospital**

Pediatric SSHO _____

Name _____

### Pain behaviour/signs

eg crying, screaming, moaning in distress
*Please note time, duration and nature of pain behaviours
along with heart rate and what helped.*

↓

### Initial comfort measures

eg reposition, massage feet, put music on, check if pad needs
changing, mouth care, etc.

↓

If still displaying pain behaviours after initial comfort measures try
### Paracetamol 500mg

↓

If still displaying pain behaviours 30 mins after initial comfort
measures and Paracetamol, try further comfort measures and
### Codeine phosphate 15mg

↓

If still displaying pain behaviours one hour after first dose of codeine
try further comfort measures and second dose of
### Codeine phosphate 15mg
*Max 2 doses codeine per 8 hours, max 4 doses per 24 hours.*

↓

If still distressed one hour after second dose of codeine and comfort
measures call doctor for further advice.
If *after hours* call link nurse and consider transfer to hospital.


**Note**: If repeated episodes ask doctor to consider regular analgesia
(eg regular Paracetamol for next week)


School nurse _____

SHO/doctor _____

# 10 Partnerships with parents and children

It is easy for families and children to become lost in the complexities of policies and protocols, legal requirements and health and safety guidance. Working in partnership with parents and children can help to ensure that policies remain focussed on children and their needs.

Good communication with families is essential to building a partnership and should be at the centre of an inclusion policy for children with complex health needs.

### How can partnership with parents be achieved?

- Information for parents should be written in clear plain language. Bolton's early years leaflet for parents is included at the end of this chapter as an example.
- Schools and other settings should promote policies of openness which will encourage parents to share information about their children's health needs
- Parents should be invited to attend and participate in meetings, reviews, risk assessments and training relating to their children. An example from the Scarborough, Whitby and Ryedale Trust is included to illustrate the importance of building trust and confidence with parents.

*All the exemplars demonstrate the involvement of parents at meetings, reviews and training sessions.*

**example** *James has unstable diabetes. At the age of three years he was due to start at nursery. His mother and the nursery staff were extremely anxious. The nursery is attached to a school which managed older children with straight forward diabetes well. They felt James was different, but they were prepared to try.*

*The head teacher and community paediatrician got together, with the child's mother, grandmother, nursery teacher, school special educational needs co-ordinator, nursery teaching assistant, the specialist nurse for diabetes and the school secretary, who is a first aider.*

*Over a cup of tea in the staff room the group worked together on writing up the health care plan. As the detailed information was discussed, the nurse for diabetes showed everyone how to check blood sugars and each person had a go at doing this. The meeting discussed the upper and lower safe levels, which were already established. James played on the floor of the staff room until he got bored and then was taken into nursery for an introductory visit.*

*Once the health care plan was typed up, a copy was sent to everyone who attended the meeting.*

*The result of involving the family and staff in this way was that the mother and the school felt happier and more confident about James starting at the nursery.*

- Schools and other settings should be open and honest with parents about their limitations. Service providers and families need a common understanding of what can be managed and how it will be managed. Parents can choose to manage risk in many ways but some of these options will not be open to service providers.

## How can partnerships with children and young people be achieved?

Legislation and guidance requires agencies to ensure that children and young people are consulted and participate in decisions that affect their lives. The SEN Code of Practice (2001) states:

> *All children should be involved in making decisions where possible right from the start of their education ... Participation in education is a process that will necessitate children being given the opportunity to make choices and to understand that their views matter. (p.28)*

The following can help to build partnerships with children and young people:
- Children and young people should be encouraged to take as much responsibility as they are able for their own health needs and the decisions relating to those needs

*Exemplar 1 (Kamahl) demonstrates the decision Kamahl made to receive his feed in the dinning room with his class mates.*

- Children and young people should attend and participate in meetings and reviews held to discuss their health needs
- The dignity and privacy of children and young people should be respected at all times. An idea which came out of the research conducted by York University (Mukherjee, S et al, 2000) was the use of 'smart cards'. Smart cards are held by the young people and include their name and other information they may wish to disclose quickly or discretely to teachers about their condition.

*Exemplar 3 (Anita) demonstrates good practice with regard to dignity and privacy.*

- Policies and practice should recognise that all children regardless of the severity of their disabilities can communicate, and the people working with them should find ways of enabling them to do so. All paperwork should include a section on the child's views. As a minimum requirement it should state how the child indicates both happiness and distress.

This last point is particularly important for children who are unable to communicate using language or signing, but who communicate in a unique way through their emotional responses. A 'communication passport' carried by the child helps ensure a more child-centred approach.

Communication passports include information about the child, how they communicate and how to interpret their communication. An example of a communication guide is included at the end of this chapter. Further information of the development of passport is included in the Resource section at the end of this handbook.

---

Included at the end of this chapter are:

**10.1** Leaflet for parents on medicines developed by Bolton early years team

**10.2** Communication passport – SENAPS, Essex County Council

## Summary

Items of medication in UNLABELLED containers WILL NOT be accepted.

Items of ILLEGIBLY LABELLED MEDICATION WILL NOT BE ADMINISTERED.

You MUST provide complete WRITTEN AND SIGNED instructions for ALL medication.

5

**earlyyears & CHILDCARE TEAM**

This leaflet has been adapted from the guidance document for 'Supporting pupils with medical needs'.

Produced by
- Val Packer, SEN Advisory Teacher (IMPACT)
- Bolton NHS Primary Care Trust
- Karen Evans, Hospital/ Home Teaching Service

6

Setting logo

# Administration of medication

## Summary guidance for parents/carers

*For use in non-maintained settings*

---

## Administration of medication in nursery

To ensure the SAFE administration of medication in the setting, the following guidelines have been produced.

If these guidelines are NOT followed then unfortunately the medication CANNOT be given.

Please note: the room leader/authorised person can administer Calpol/ Paracetamol which is not prescribed by a doctor when authorised by a parent/carer. Staff will always ring parents first to confirm.

Items of medication in unlabelled containers will not be accepted.

2

## Guidelines to be followed

1 Parents/carers are responsible for providing the Manager with adequate information regarding their child's condition and medication.

2 It is the parents/carers responsibility to inform nursery in writing when the medication is discontinued or the dosage changed.

3 Medication WILL NOT be accepted in nursery without complete written and signed instruction. Parents/carers should sign when they have left or collected medicines. Ideally medicine bottles should be marked with levels to indicate how much has been used at home.

3

4 ONLY reasonable quantities of medication should be supplied to nursery, e.g. a maximum of 4 weeks supply at any one time.

5 Each item of medication must be delivered in the original container and handed directly to the Manager or Room Leader.

6 Parents/carers are responsible for the collection of medicines

Each container MUST be clearly labelled with the following:
- Pupil's name
- Name of medication
- Dosage
- Frequency of dosage
- Date of dispensing
- Storage requirements (if important)
- Expiry date

4

**Example of Fred's pen portrait, prepared by Fred and his carers and teacher (This pen portrait could be written in the 'third person')**

I am 8 years old.

I am usually happy and contented and able to show adults who know me when I am uncomfortable, sad or in pain. I love people talking to me and I can recognise familiar voices. My movements can be a bit uncontrolled. I only have very limited vision so I rely on my hearing and my ability to touch to make sense of where I am and what I should be doing. I need help to be able to move from one position to another and will try and help in movement activity. Sometimes I get uncomfortable so moving me and helping me change my posture including my sitting or standing position makes me feel better. I will smile if I'm OK.

I enjoy being cuddled and reach out to touch faces and hair. I like to try and find objects that are within my reach and I can anticipate a simple, noisy cause and effect activity. I love being free to wriggle around on the mat and I stop moving when I hear a sound or feel a touch. I enjoy standing in my supportive standing frame and I can take some weight through my feet when closely supported by someone who knows me well. When I sit in my supportive seating chair I am able to hold my head up better and also reach for an activity and use both my hands. I can get quite tired very quickly and then I need extra help to hold my head up or I need a rest.

Due to my very sensitive mouth, I have difficulty eating and drinking and have a 'tummy peg' to make sure I have enough food and drink. I have severe epileptic fits. My health care plans support both these medical needs. I am totally dependent on adults for my personal care.

**Example of the goals and aspirations illustrating the person centred approach to planning to child and family focused planning**

1 Fred to be able to make himself understood to unfamiliar adults so that he can broaden his circle of support and his carers can be more confident about other people looking after and caring for him
2 Fred to be able to make some choices in what he would like to do so that he learns how to make decisions
3 Fred to be able to stand, with adult support, so he can help with his mobility
4 Fred to be able to take an active role in his personal and self help skills
5 Fred to be able to activate a wide variety of cause and effect toys so that he expands his opportunities for play
6 Fred's carers wish to be able to look after Fred at home for as long as possible

| Goals | What is happening now | People involved in helping Fred and his carers | Actions | Monitor and review – including time scales and dates and the opportunity for all involved to contribute |
|---|---|---|---|---|
| 1. Fred to be able to make himself understood to unfamiliar adults | Fred is able to make himself understood by adults who know him very well | Carers, teachers, key worker, SaLT, OT, short break and shared carers, family support workers, sessional workers at the local activity clubs | Joint re-assessment by SaLT, teacher and carers | SaLT, teacher and key worker every term. Frequent recording |
| 2. Fred to be able to make choices | Fred is able to make a few choices by demonstrating, to familiar adults, whether he likes or dislikes an activity | Carers, teachers, key worker, OT, SaLT, short break and shared carers, family support workers, sessional workers at local activity clubs | Joint re-assessment by SaLT, OT, teacher and carer | Teacher, SaLT, key worker every term. Frequent recording |
| 3. Fred to be able to stand, with adult support | Fred is able to stand momentarily, with maximum adult support | Carers, PT, teacher, key workers, family support workers, short break workers, shared carers | Re-assessment and teaching for selected staff and carers by PT | Teacher, PT and OT. Episode of direct intervention every half term PT. Orthotics every term (PT) |
| 4. Fred to be able to take an active role in his personal care and self help skills | Fred is sensitive to having a spoon or toothbrush in his mouth and requires maximum support for all personal care including eating and drinking activities. He is 'tummy peg' fed | Carers, teachers, specialist nurses, dietician, SaLT, OT, dental hygienist, key worker, short break and shared carers, family support workers | Review de-sensitising programme – SaLT, OT | Team around the child, every half term co-ordinated by school nurse |
| 5. Fred to be able to activate a wide variety of cause and effect toys | Fred is able to play with two familiar cause and effect toys | Carers, teachers, key workers, OT, family support workers, short break, shared carers and sessional workers at local activity clubs | Update from OT, positioning for being able to use hands | Teacher, OT and key worker every term. Frequent recording |
| 6. Fred's carers to be able to look after him at home for as long as possible | Carers require support from short break, shared carers and family support workers. Carers have many disturbed nights. Carers not confident about holiday activities | Social worker, short break and shared carers, family support workers, sessional workers at local activity clubs | Referral to doctor for further advice | Practical support arrangements reviewed as per LAC regulations. Monitor of sleep patterns – every half term – parent and teacher/key worker |

| Key skills | Component skill | Key objectives or learning targets | Evidence of success | Strategies to support |
|---|---|---|---|---|
| Personal and social | Personal | To define a positive 'no' response | Demonstrates the positive 'no' response to familiar adults who reinforce the response | Communication passport |
| | Social | To actively participate in group activities with familiar and unfamiliar people | Consistently holding or lifting up his head and/or smiling/vocalising movement when called by his name even if he does not recognise the voice | Posture and movement |
| Communication | Speaking | To be able to demonstrate a definite 'no' which is accurately interpreted by an unfamiliar adult | Unfamiliar adults, such as a different family support worker is able to accurately interpret a negative response from Fred | Communication Communication passport |
| Etc | | | | |

*Page 2* **Fred to be able to make choices**

| Key skills | Component skill | Key objectives or learning targets | Evidence of success | Strategies to support |
|---|---|---|---|---|
| Communication | Speaking | To begin to communicate choices by eye pointing and smiling/making happy vocalisations sounds | Smiles and keeps smiling when eye pointing to a chosen activity/toy which he can then participate in | Communication Communication passport |
| | Listening | To begin to respond to some key words within the context of very familiar routines | Smiles and vocalises to the names of familiar people | |
| Mathematics | Measures and shapes | To explore different objects placed within his reach | Moving his hands to touch and knock wobbly sounding toys | Posture and movement |
| | Making sense of problems | To feel a range of substances and materials and begin to discriminate between them | Keeping his hands on soft gentle materials whilst moving his hands away from harsh materials | Posture and movement |
| Problem solving | | To anticipate certain actions and effects | Shows excitement when waiting for a toy to make a noise or move | |
| Physical | Manipulation | To purposefully feel and touch objects | Reaching out and exploring objects | Posture and movement |

*Page 3* **Fred to be able to stand with adult support**

| Key skills | Component skill | Key objectives or learning targets | Evidence of success | Strategies to support |
|---|---|---|---|---|
| Physical | Movement | To be able to take some weight through his legs when supported by a familiar adult | Taking weight through his legs when transferring from his wheelchair to a chair | Daily stands in the supportive standing frame. Assisted supported standing. Posture and movement. Moving and therapeutic handling |
| | | To be able to bridge | Bridging whilst lying on the mat | Posture and movement. PE schemes of work |
| | | To be able to freely kick his legs | Kicking a large light ball with R and L feet whilst lying on the mat or sitting with support | PE schemes of work |
| Etc | | | | |

*Page 4* **Fred to be able to take an active role in his personal care and self help skill**

| Key skills | Component skill | Key objectives or learning targets | Evidence of success | Strategies to support |
|---|---|---|---|---|
| Physical | Movement | To be able to assist in personal care by 'bridging' | Actively bridging at each personal care session | Posture and movement |
| | Manipulation | To be able to hold feeding tube | Holding the tube during lunch and tea time feeds | Healthcare Plans |
| Communication | | To be able to indicate when thirsty | Sipping to drink from a shallow spoon after indicating he is thirsty by sticking his tongue out | Feeding and drinking |
| | | To tolerate having his teeth cleaned | Keeping his head still and his mouth relaxed when it is teeth cleaning time | De sensitising programme |
| Personal and social | Personal | To be able to recognise 'object of reference' | Routinely holding the appropriate object of reference | Posture and movement. Communication passport |
| | | To assist with removing coat | Holding sleeve of coat to help | Posture and movement |

| Key skills | Component skill | Key objectives or learning targets | Evidence of success | Strategies to support |
|---|---|---|---|---|
| ICT | Modelling and control | To be able to operate a variety of touch switch toys | Lifting hands and placing on switch and smiling at the effect with familiar toys, and lifting and placing hands on the same switch but activating a different toy and developing an awareness of the difference | Posture and movement. Communication |
| Study skills | Concentration | To become less reliant on adult support when playing with switch toys | Switching cause and effect toys off and on, smiling at the effect and repeating action independent of adults | |
| Physical | Manipulation | To be able to relax his hands and place them on a switch | Placing his hands purposefully onto a switch with minimal adult prompt | Posture and movement. Communication |
| Etc | | | | |

*Page 6* **Fred's carers to be able to look after him at home for as long as possible**

| Key skills | Evidence of success | Strategies to support |
|---|---|---|
| Fred's carers to consistently have undisturbed nights | Fred sleeps through the night | School timetable to support regular rest periods, activities after lunch and morning hydro sessions to encourage Fred to stay awake all day. Taxi to have a supply of Fred's favourite music tapes. Structured bedtime routine and healthcare plans in place. Fred to have sleep system (posture support) |
| Fred's carers to receive short breaks | Fred's practical support arrangements are in place and reviewed regularly | Practical support arrangements: • 20 nights of short break arrangements • 7.30 until 8.30 family support x3 days a week, term time • One Saturday in a month shared care |
| Fred's carers to feel confident about Fred attending the local activity group | Fred is able to communicate simple needs through his communication passport | Communication passport. Posture and movement/Moving and therapeutic handling. Healthcare Plans |

## Example of a quick reference guide

Prepared by parents/carers, teacher/plan operator and the team around the child *(ensure there are links to the goals and skills to be learned)*

| Encourage | Discourage |
| --- | --- |
| Sitting on the mat with my legs crossed with support from an adult | Slumping against support from an adult with both my legs twisted |
| Sitting straight in my chair | Twisting my head in my chair |
| Holding my head up and playing with activities with my hands | Putting my head on my hands and biting my knuckles |
| Making me choose what toys I want to play with | Just giving me the same toys to play with |

## Example of a communication guide

Prepared by parents/carers, teacher/plan operator and the 'team around the child'

| When I do this | People think I mean | You should do |
| --- | --- | --- |
| Smile | I am saying 'yes'. I am happy. I like what I am doing. | Give me time to smile and act according to my answer of 'yes'. |
| Lift up my left hand and bang the tray (I am just learning to do this) | I am trying to say 'no'. | Ask me the question again and act according to my answer of 'no'. |
| Close my eyes and moan | I am uncomfortable. I am sad. I am bored. I don't like what I am doing. | 1. Ask me if I am uncomfortable, if I smile, move my position, for example, if I am in my wheelchair – take me out and let me stretch out on a mat. If I'm on the mat, sit me back into my chair See my practical support plans to help you do this properly. 2. If I don't smile, just talk to me and see if you can cheer me up. 3. If I don't smile, see if I would like to do something else, offer me a choice. |
| Keep letting my head fall forwards | I am tired. | Let me rest, stretched out on the mat, or in my side lying board. |
| Stick my tongue out | I am thirsty. | Give me a little warm drink of water from my special mug. See my practical support plans to help you do this properly. |
| Cry but there are no tears | I am cross. | Check to see if I need anything, change my activity or include me in an activity. Move me from sitting next to someone who may upsetting me. |
| Screw up my hands | I feel very unsafe. | Give me more support and help. |
| Screw my nose up and twist my head | I have got a tummy ache. | Help me change my position. Give me sips of warm water to drink |

# Appendix 1
# Exemplars

All the exemplars are based upon real-life case examples, but have been altered and anonymised in order to respect the confidentiality of parties involved.

### Exemplar 1 **Kamahl**

Kamahl aged seven years is in Year 2 at Grove Lodge School. The school has 170 pupils on its roll and there are 28 pupils in Kamahl's class. He has had problems of food intolerance from an early age, particularly with dairy products. He was born prematurely, had severe gastro-oesophageal reflux as a baby and as a result of a combination of nutritional problems, he has had a gastrostomy for overnight feeding since the age of three years. He has a low-profile gastrostomy button.

Before Kamahl joined the school, his parents met with the headteacher, school nurse and community children's nurse in order to consider his possible health care needs. Kamahl has had a health care plan since he joined the school in the reception class. His gastrostomy has presented no problems whatsoever since he commenced school.

His weight has always been around the third centile, but has recently been falling below that level. Kamahl's mother prepares a lunch time meal and snacks to be brought into school each day, but he does not eat well at school (or at home) and it has recently been decided to introduce a bolus gastrostomy feed at lunch time. It will take approximately 30 minutes to administer his feed.

Kamahl's mother informed the school of this change in his regime and a 'planning' meeting was held at the school attended by:
- Mr and Mrs Ahmad, Kamahl's mother and father
- school nurse
- community children's nurse
- community dietician
- headteacher
- class teacher
- special educational needs coordinator
- meal time support assistant (MSA)

At the meeting, it was agreed that the community children's nurse (CCN) would accompany Mrs Ahmad to provide a programme of training and assessment of competence for the MSA who has expressed an interest in administering Kamahl's lunch time feed. The programme of training will take place over a five day period, with either Mrs Ahmad or the CCN (or both) attending the school at lunch time each day to train/supervise the MSA.

Kamahl has asked that he receive his feed in the dining room with his class mates. He says that all his friends know about his 'special' button and he has told them that he will be having a 'special' feed at lunch time.

It has been agreed that Mrs Ahmad will bring a week's worth of supplies into school each Monday morning. These are to be kept in a sports holdall with a padlock which the family have provided. The sports holdall will be stored in a cupboard in the school office.

Kamahl's feed is pre-packaged (in tins) and needs to be transferred into a feeding dispenser which connects via a flexible tubing to his gastrostomy tube. The feeding 'kit' is assembled in the multi-purpose room adjacent to the school office [At other times the room is used for school medicals and minor treatments – it is also a storage area for a variety of school equipment.] The room has a sink with hot and cold running water and a 'clean area' has been identified where preparation of Kamahl's feed can be undertaken.

Once the feed has been transferred into the feeding 'kit', it is taken to Kamahl in the dining room and he receives his feed, with discrete supervision, whilst sitting with his class mates. As part of the procedure, the gastrostomy site is discretely observed, the patency of the gastrostomy tube is checked and the tube is flushed with cooled, boiled water before and after administering the feed.

The MSA watched Mrs Ahmad and the CCN prepare the feed for administration on Monday and Tuesday. On Wednesday she administered the feed under supervision from the CCN and on Thursday she felt confident to both prepare the feed for administration and to give the feed – with Mrs Ahmad supervising. The training programme was based upon an existing local health Trust protocol developed by the CCN team for training parents and has been adapted for school use. The protocol includes several aspects of gastrostomy care including:
- hand washing procedure
- preparing the feed for administration
- observation of the gastrostomy site
- confirming the patency of the gastrostomy tube
- flushing the gastrostomy, before and after the feed
- administration of the feed
- care, cleansing and disposal of equipment
- troubleshooting guide

The protocol included a section in which Mrs Ahmad, the CCN and the MSA all provided signed, dated confirmation of the content of the training programme that had been delivered, as well as details of the supporting documentation/information that had been provided to the MSA during the course of the training. In addition, the CCN confirmed that she had assessed the competence of the MSA to undertake the procedures set out in the protocol and also provided details of the arrangements for on-going monitoring of the MSA's competence. A copy of the protocol is to be kept with Kamahl's feeding equipment, and a second copy has been appended to his health care plan.

All of this documentation was 'signed off' on Friday, the fifth day of the training programme and the MSA took over Kamahl's care the following Monday.

The CCN agreed to attend the school once per week for the first month and provided an air-call bleep contact number and a commitment to attend the school should any problems arise.

A number of policy documents have been considered/consulted in relation to Kamahl's care in school including:
- infection control
- storage of medicines/medical equipment
- clinical safety/emergencies risk assessment
- disposal of clinical waste
- consent to treatment
- safeguarding children
- confidentiality

The school health and safety officer has confirmed that the arrangements which have been put in place to support Kamahl in school comply with the relevant sections of each of the policies.

Kamahl's health care plan has been amended to incorporate the changes to his lunch time regime.

*Mark Whiting, Consultant Nurse,*
*Children with Complex Health Needs,*
*Hertfordshire Partnership NHS Trust*


## Exemplar 2  Gareth

Gareth is four years old and is scheduled to join his local primary school in the reception class. He was born at 28 weeks gestation, spent the first ten weeks of his life in hospital and as a result of being ventilated as a neonate has developed a narrowing of his airway. He required a tracheostomy to support his breathing when he was only a few weeks old in order to maintain his airway and this has remained in place ever since.

His growth and development have been otherwise unremarkable and despite his prematurity, he is both cognitively and physically on a par with his peers, though his airway remains a major cause for concern.

In order for Gareth to be safe he needs to be accompanied by an adult who is skilled in all aspects of tracheostomy care at all times. He requires regular suctioning via his tracheostomy in order to maintain his airway. If his tracheostomy becomes blocked this would be considered as a medical emergency and the tracheostomy tube would need to be replaced promptly.

Prior to starting school, Gareth has been cared for at home by his parents who learned to care for his tracheostomy when it was first created. He has not attended nursery school. His family receive support and guidance from the local team of Children's Community Nurses. In advance of Gareth starting school a planning meeting was set up to ensure that all of Gareth's needs could be met effectively and that his transition into education was seamless. The meeting involved:
- Gareth's parents
- children's community nurse (CCN)
- headteacher
- classroom teacher
- special educational needs co-ordinator
- school nurse

The planning meeting highlighted that in order to ensure Gareth's safety a support worker should be employed to meet his health care needs in school. It was agreed that comprehensive risk assessment should be undertaken jointly by the school and the health care professionals.

The planning meeting took place in the summer term prior to Gareth starting school, in order to ensure that adequate time was available to advertise, recruit and train the support care worker for Gareth to commence school in the autumn. This also allowed adequate time for a comprehensive risk assessment to be completed.

It was agreed at the planning meeting that the support worker should be employed and managed by the school – a joint funding arrangement was agreed between the local education authority and the National Health Service (local primary care trust). It was additionally agreed that the one-to-one support worker would be trained and assessed by the CCN and Gareth's mother during the Summer holiday in order that he/she would be fully prepared in time for the beginning of the new school year. The training programme used to prepare and assess the support worker was adapted from one used by the NHS Trust and the CCN team to train other respite carers. It included the following aspects of tracheostomy care:
- hand washing procedure
- principals of suction and practical suctioning skills for a tracheostomy

- observation of the tracheostomy site
- observation and recognition of changes in breathing and blocked tracheostomy
- changing the tracheostomy tube both routinely and in an emergency.
- basic life support (BLS)
- care, cleansing and disposal of equipment
- troubleshooting guide

The CCN agreed to attend the school once per week for the first month and provided an air-call bleep contact number and a commitment to attend the school should any problems arise. The support worker's competence would be monitored and formally re-assessed on a six-monthly basis in the first instance. In addition, she would be provided with annual updates on basic life support and tracheostomy competencies. The training programme documentation included a section in which Gareth's parents, the CCN and the support worker all provided signed, dated confirmation of the content of the training programme that had been delivered, as well as details of the supporting documentation/ information that had been provided to the support worker during the course of the training. A competency framework was also included.

The risk assessment addressed the following issues:
- It was not necessary for any specific adaptations to be made to the school as he was fully mobile and would be able to access all areas of the school and all aspects of the curriculum.
- An area close to the classroom was identified where the support worker would be able to wash his/her hands on a regular basis in order to adhere to good hand-washing practise and reduce the risk of cross infection.
- A separate closed-lid waste bin was purchased to ensure that clinical waste such as suction catheters and gloves could be segregated from the other general rubbish in the classroom and disposed of safely.
- A weekly clinical waste collection was set up with the local council in order that the waste was removed appropriately, and a lockable waste storage area was designated to house the used bags prior to collection.
- A power supply to charge Gareth's portable suction machine was also identified to ensure that Gareth's suction machine was always in full functioning order.
- An area to store equipment supplies was identified in the school office to ensure that adequate suction equipment was available and provision for a spare suction unit to be kept in school was made to ensure that if Gareth's own machine broke down that another was available to maintain his safety.
- A discussion was held in relation to out-of-school activities and it was agreed that day trips out would not pose a problem as the carer would be able to accompany Gareth, but that if there were any trips

that were overnight that this would have to considered at the time as someone trained in Gareth's care would need to be with him 24 hours a day (the only scheduled overnight activity took place in Year 5).
- Gareth's parents agreed that they would be transporting Gareth to and from school on a daily basis, and therefore there was no need for transport provision to be arranged in this case.

A health care plan was completed for Gareth and copies of the tracheostomy care protocols and risk assessment summary were appended to this.

It was agreed that a review meeting would take place early in the autumn term and then on an annual basis. This would involve all those involved in the original pre-admission planning meeting.

A number of policy documents were considered/consulted in relation to Gareth's care in school including:
- infection control
- storage of medicines/medical equipment
- clinical safety/emergencies risk assessment
- disposal of clinical waste
- consent to treatment
- safeguarding children
- confidentiality

The school health and safety officer has confirmed that the arrangements which have been put in place to support Gareth in school comply with the relevant sections of each of the policies.

*Gaynor Evans,*
*Head of Children's Continuing Care,*
*Hertfordshire Partnership Trust*

### Exemplar 3  Anita

Anita is an active three year old identified by a mass of blonde hair, blue eyes and an inquisitive manner. She has no external features to identify her as different from her peers as developmentally and socially she is progressing appropriately for her age.

Anita's parents, Tony and Ruth, are proud of their daughter's achievements and are keen for her to commence nursery school five mornings a week. They also have a five year old daughter Ellie, who attends the infants school adjacent to the nursery and an eight month old son, Jo.

The first year of Anita's life had not been straightforward. She was born at term at the local district general hospital, but required emergency transfer to a specialist tertiary hospital for treatment of a bowel abnormality. Anita's condition was diagnosed as Hirschsprung's disease, a congenital condition in which nerve supply to part of the bowel is missing resulting in a failure of normal peristalsis and leading to enlargement of the bowel, constipation and obstruction. This represented a surgical emergency and lead to the formation of a colostomy – an opening on the surface of the abdomen whereby a portion of the colon is pulled through and attached to the skin surface. Termed as a stoma (opening), this allows waste products from the bowel to leave the body and drain into a 'stoma bag'. Anita's stoma site is situated on the lower left side of the abdomen and her collection bag is a one-piece drainable bag that includes a self-adhesive baseplate. A clipped fastening at the base of the bag allows for ease of emptying of the wet paste like consistency of Anita's bowel motion.

Anita's family were confident in her care and had established links with their local health visitor, the community children's nursing team and a specialist stoma therapist nurse who worked form the local district general hospital. Generally their contact was limited to occasions when Anita was unwell or had problems with skin care around the stoma site. The family arrange supply of their stoma bags through a GP prescription and the local chemist.

Ruth and Tony applied for Anita to start at the Peter Pan Nursery adjacent to their elder daughter Ellie's junior school. Their application was accompanied by a letter, written by themselves, outlining Anita's previous health problems and the special consideration needed for her 'toileting', or more specifically, emptying the stoma bag as required. The letter contained contact details of the local community children's nursing team (CCN) and mother's reassurance that she would wish to be involved in any teaching and training of the staff.

The school had been in contact with the family the term prior to Anita's entry and arrangements were made for the parents to attend a short pre-admission consultation with the headteacher. A subsequent appointment was then arranged after school hours for the CCN, mother and class teacher to discuss Anita's care needs in more detail. At the meeting, the CCN outlined a proposed health care plan, advising that the CCN would provide a programme of training, setting out how staff should respond if Anita's colostomy bag became unattached, or needed to be emptied. They highlighted the need for prompt action to intervene if the bag became unattached or the fastener opened so that Anita's skin did not become sore due to exposure to the waste matter and/or cause her any unnecessary upset.

The discussion included the need for Anita's privacy and appropriate changing and hand washing facilities, the provision of disposal gloves and clinical waste bags for soiled disposal products. Ruth agreed to provide a labelled changing pack with a pre-shaped colostomy bag, wipes and initial nappy bags. The nurse agreed to arrange supplies of disposal gloves, anti-bacterial hand wash/gel, collection jug and the clinical waste bags. She also arranged for the collection of the waste bags via the local council.

A training session was organised for three members of teaching staff and two support workers. A demonstration was given with a mannequin and sample stoma bags.

A health care plan was drawn up in consultation with Anita's mother. The plan confirmed that staff should be able to:
- be aware of Anita's condition
- recognise potential problems for a child with a stoma bag.
- be able to change a stoma bag efficiently and effectively.
- help maintain a healthy stoma area and keep good skin integrity around the site by cleaning appropriately.
- be aware and able to *empty* the stoma bag confidently.
- e aware of how to dispose of:
  - the contents of the bag
  - a used displaced bag
  - ask questions and practically voice their concerns

Literature from the National Advisory Service for Parents of Children with a Stoma (NASPCS) was available as a useful resource and staff kept copies of the teaching handouts in a file held in the classroom.

Upon completion of the training programme relevant staff were issued with a training protocol and a statement of training was signed and dated by the CCN, which confirmed that staff had received instruction on colostomy care, specifically based upon Anita's needs. The CCN agreed to update new staff as and when necessary and provide a revision session at the beginning of the next term.

As Anita was scheduled to be in nursery placement for a four hour session, it was agreed that the class assistant and the teacher would routinely to inspect the stoma bag at the same time that the other children were scheduled for a visit to the toilet. If necessary the stoma bag would emptied. An area of the toilet/washroom was identified for storage of waste disposal bags and gloves. A prepared bag containing necessary supplies was kept on Anita's coat peg and she brought this to the toilet herself. Anita preferred to stand whilst stoma care was undertaken and she complied well with assistance. Anita was familiar with her own routine and could also ask for 'bag care' if she felt uncomfortable. Her familiarity with one specific 'helper' was identified. The nursery staff were made aware that Anita's urinary function was normal and therefore, if she needed the toilet, she alerted staff so her bag could be checked at the same time.

During the first few days Ruth arranged to stay on site as a helper, offering assistance with Anita's checks and care as required. Once Anita was settled, and the staff felt confident and competent to supervise her care, Ruth withdrew and family telephone contact numbers were provided in case required. The Community Children's Nurses also left contact numbers and agreed to be available to attend the school if it was needed. During the first term Ruth was contacted once when Anita was upset and insisted on her mother's presence.

A number of policy documents have been considered/consulted in relation to Anita's care in nursery, these include:
- infection control – including hand washing
- clinical safety/emergencies risk assessment
- disposal of clinical waste
- consent to treatment
- safeguarding children
- confidentiality

The headteacher and the named health and safety officer have subsequently confirmed that the arrangements have been put in place to support Anita in nursery and currently comply with the above named policies.

Anita is fully integrated into all activities with the nursery day. She currently does not require additional help, though present arrangements will be reviewed next term when Anita will be assessed in line with application to join the reception class on a full-time basis.

### Reference

*National Advisory Service for Parents of Children with a Stoma*
John Malcolm (Chairman), 51 Anderston Drive, Valley View Park, Darnel, Ayrshire KA17 0DG

*Janette Harrison, Modern Matron,*
*Children's Community and Specialist Practice,*
*Hertfordshire Partnership NHS Trust*

### Exemplar 4  **Daniel**

Daniel is 11 years old and is in Year 6 at Redvers Primary School which has 180 pupils on its roll. He is due to start at St John's Secondary School in September this year. Daniel has spina bifida. He has good upper limb strength and function, but he has reduced muscle strength and sensation in his legs. He has a slight scoliosis (curvature) of the spine, which is under regular review at the local orthopaedic hospital. He wears Ankle Foot Orthoses (AFOs – foot splints) every day to support and maintain his ankles in a good position.

Daniel is able to sit independently. He uses a pair of crutches when walking. His walking distance is becoming increasingly restricted by painful muscle contractures and calluses of his feet. Consequently, Daniel is spending significant periods of time in a self-propelled wheelchair, in which he has been practising independent wheelchair skills for the last six months at his present school. As a result of perceptual and spatial awareness difficulties, he is not yet competent with his wheelchair with regards to road safety and awareness, or in negotiating a range of obstacles including narrow spaces such as doorways and corridors.

St John's School has 1200 pupils and is on a large site, with a main building of three storeys and separate science labs. Daniel is feeling extremely anxious about the prospect of moving to a larger school and meeting new people.

During the summer term before he is due to transfer, a meeting takes place to discuss Daniel's needs at his new school to ensure a smooth transition. It is attended by:

- Daniel
- his mother
- present class teacher
- present learning support assistant
- secondary school special educational needs co-ordinator
- Year 7 head
- occupational therapist
- physiotherapist
- secondary school nurse

At the meeting, concerns are raised regarding Daniel's limited mobility and his wheelchair skills. The occupational therapist informs the meeting that Daniel is to attend a wheelchair course during the summer holidays to address his wheelchair manoeuvrability skills. The physiotherapist reports that Daniel is able to walk short distances and negotiate stairs with the use of crutches. However, he would be vulnerable in crowded corridors and stairs, and would find the negotiation of heavy doors difficult. It is agreed that Daniel will be allowed to leave lessons two minutes before the bell goes, with a friend, to allow him time to reach his next lesson safely. Daniel's friend would need to carry his bag for him as Daniel's balance would be affected if he carried it himself.

Concerns are raised as to how Daniel would access the upper floors of the school should Daniel's mobility deteriorate further, causing him to be unable to negotiate the stairs. It is suggested that either his lessons could be timetabled to take place on the ground floor, or that the school applies to have a lift installed in the main building to access the upper floors. It is agreed that this would need ongoing review, taking into consideration changes in Daniel's skills.

It is recognised that Daniel would be vulnerable should there be a need for an emergency evacuation (for instance in case of fire) as Daniel is unable to propel his wheelchair quickly and safely. It is agreed that Daniel should be pushed in his wheelchair by the teacher taking the present class if the evacuation takes place in lessons, or by the supervising teacher on playground duty should the evacuation take place during break times. Should Daniel be on an upper floor and unable to use the stairs safely during an evacuation procedure, there should be a designated safe area clearly marked where he can wait for the fire personnel to rescue him. The fire personnel should be consulted by the school with regards to the planning of the designated safe area.

On school outings, Daniel would need to take his crutches and his wheelchair. He would require using his wheelchair for distances further than 500 metres. Should there be residential school trips, including going abroad, every effort must be made to include Daniel in the trip, with any relevant risk assessments carried out to ensure his needs are met, and to ensure his safety.

During a tour of the school site, it is noted that the benches in the science labs would be too high for Daniel to access from his wheelchair. It is proposed that the school purchases a height adjustable table for Daniel to use in science lessons.

The physiotherapist informs the meeting that Daniel has a standing frame which he uses in his present school. This allows Daniel to have a sustained stretch in standing, whilst still being able to participate in lessons and access the curriculum. It is agreed that this arrangement can continue at his new school. It is agreed that the school will identify an area of safe storage for the standing frame during nights and weekends. The physiotherapist will arrange a visit to the school at the start of the autumn term to show Daniel's teaching staff how to place him in the standing frame correctly and safely. The school would need to carry out a manual handling risk assessment of their staff with regards to the procedure of assisting Daniel in and out of the standing frame. Currently, Daniel is able to step in and out of the standing frame, however his mobility may deteriorate in the coming years, and he may require hoisted assistance in and out of the standing frame. Should this happen, the school staff would need to attend manual handling training sessions in order to ensure proficiency in the use of a hoist and standing sling.

The physiotherapist reports that at present, Daniel has a stretching programme that is carried out in his current school by the learning support assistant, who has been comprehensively trained by the physiotherapist. There was some discussion as to whether it would continue to be appropriate to be carried out in the secondary school, as it would emphasise Daniel's physical difficulties in comparison to his peer group. It is suggested that the physiotherapist review Daniel's stretching programme with Daniel and his mother in order that the stretches be undertaken at home. Daniel feels that this would be much better.

The occupational therapist reports that Daniel would require assistance carrying books, scientific apparatus, etc in the classroom, and carrying his tray at mealtimes, due to his being unable to carry objects when using his crutches or propelling himself in his wheelchair. The Year 7 head agrees to liaise with all Daniel's subject teachers with regards to encouraging his classmates to assist him when necessary.

With regards to toileting, Daniel performs intermittent catheterisation independently and therefore requires access to a suitably equipped disabled toilet with clinical waste disposal facilities.

Daniel should be encouraged to participate in PE lessons with his peers. He would be able to participate in team sports such as basketball in his wheelchair. The PE staff would need to consider adapting the PE curriculum to meet Daniel's abilities. The physiotherapist would be willing for the PE staff to consult her with regards to making adaptations and stating what Daniel is able to do and what he is unable to do, to ensure maximum integration.

A number of policy documents have been considered with regards to Daniel's care in school, including:
- emergencies/risk assessment
- moving and handling
- disposal of clinical waste
- consent to treatment
- safeguarding children
- confidentiality

The meeting concludes with the formulation of an agreed action plan, signed by all present. A health care plan will be written and distributed to the relevant professionals, Daniel and his mother, to agree to the plan which will be in place when he commences Year 7.

*Lucy Wills and Karen Woollard,*
*Community Children's Physiotherapists,*
*Hertfordshire Partnership Trust*

### Exemplar 5   Bethan

Bethan, aged 14, attends a local school for children with profound and multiple learning disabilities. She was diagnosed HIV positive when she was four years old, after contracting cryptococcal meningitis. She was extremely sick, required ventilation in hospital for several weeks and made a slow recovery. As a result of the meningitis she was left with some auditory and significant neurological impairment. She is prescribed antiretroviral therapy for her HIV infection.

She lives with her mother and two sisters. Bethan's mother, Grace, has symptomatic HIV infection though both sisters are negative. Grace was initially extremely reluctant to share information about Bethan's HIV status with members of the professional network. When Bethan first came to the school the only people aware of her HIV status were the school nurses, community paediatrician and the community children's nurse. Grace has been treated for depression and is currently on anti-depressants and being monitored by a community psychiatric nurse.

Bethan uses an alternative and augmentative communication device both at home and in school. She has a limited understanding of her health problems. She is aware that she attends hospitals and knows her doctors and nurses but is not aware of her diagnosis. She has a good relationship with her teacher and music therapist within the school.

The school nurse considered a number of policy documents in relation to Bethan's care within the school. These included:
- confidentiality
- infection control
- consent to treatment
- safeguarding children
- clinical safety/emergencies risk assessment
- disposal of clinical waste

Following concern about Bethan's adherence with medication and her increasingly difficult behaviour, the community children's nurse called a meeting, which was attended by:
- Grace
- school nurse
- community children's nurse
- community psychiatric nurse
- consultant paediatrician

The aim of the meeting was to explore how best to provide support in managing Bethan's medication regime and provide emotional support for Bethan, whose behaviour had deteriorated in the previous term. Grace had shared how difficult it was to get Bethan to take her medicines as she was clamping her teeth, refusing to swallow, and spitting. It was agreed that as her treatment was now daily the school nurses and community children's nurses could take on this task in order to support Grace, as the community psychiatric nurse felt this was compounding Grace's depression and having a negative impact on Grace and Bethan's relationship.

During the meeting, consideration was given to possible disclosure of diagnosis to Bethan and key professionals within the school. It was felt by all that in order for Bethan to be told her diagnosis it would be necessary to include the teacher and music therapist as they could offer the best support for Bethan. Grace agreed and gave her consent that key professionals within the school should be aware of Bethan's HIV diagnosis. Awareness of this diagnosis would enable a more appropriate health care plan to be developed within the school

It was decided at this meeting that the team of key professionals should include:
- headteacher
- class teacher
- music therapist
- physiotherapist
- community paediatrician
- community children's nurse
- school nurse

It was felt that the community psychiatric nurse was not required to attend these meetings as Grace had established a good relationship with both the community children's nurse and the school nurse, and that they could support Grace during this time. The CPN would be made aware of discussions held and action plans in order to provide on-going psychological care for Grace.

As a result of this second meeting it was agreed that with respect to key policies:
- **Confidentiality** This would be conducted on a strict need to know basis. If it was felt that for the benefit of Bethan's educational, psychological and physical well-being others should be informed, this would first be discussed with Grace and her consent obtained.
- **Infection control/disposal of clinical waste** Universal precautions are adhered to within the school at all times. Grace will be informed of any community acquired infections or outbreaks e.g. chicken pox within the school, in order to minimize risk to Bethan due to her compromised immune function.
- **Consent to treatment** The care plan involved the school nurse administering Bethan's medication on a daily basis. Grace agreed to supply the school with Bethan's antiretroviral medications, which are to be stored in a locked cupboard in the medical room.
- **Safeguarding children** In light of Bethan's health needs, behaviour and her mothers depression it was decided Bethan was not at risk but fulfilled the criteria of a child in need. Therefore it was felt that extra support at this time would be a positive intervention. The most appropriate person within the school setting was identified as the music therapist. Weekly sessions were timetabled for the current term. These would be reviewed at the next review meeting.

It was also decided that the class teacher and the community children's nurse would undertake a collaborative piece of work with Bethan around disclosure of her diagnosis. This would initially involve discussions about the body and how it functions and then develop into a more detailed interaction about Bethan's illness. Bethan would be made aware which professionals knew in order to make her feel more secure about her situation.

On conclusion of this meeting, the agreed action plan was documented and signed by all relevant participants. To protect confidentiality this document was to be kept separate to Bethan's school records and in a locked filing cabinet accessible only to the headteacher

*Wendy Faulknall, Manager, Community Children's Nursing Team, Queen Elizabeth Hospital, Woolwich, London*

# Appendix 2
# Legal framework

This appendix sets out the legal framework for schools and local education authorities in the management of medicines and complex health needs in schools and early years settings.

It is to be noted that this advice does not constitute an authoritative legal interpretation of the provisions of any enactments or regulations or the common law: that is exclusively a matter for the courts. It remains for authorities, schools and settings to develop their policies in the light of their statutory responsibilities and their own assessment of local needs and resources.

### General background

1 Local authorities, schools and governing bodies are responsible for the health and safety of pupils in their care. The legal framework for schools dealing with the health and safety of *all* their pupils derives from health and safety legislation. The law imposes duties on employers. Primary care trusts (PCTs) and NHS Trusts also have legal responsibilities for the health of residents in their area.

2 The registered person in early years settings, which can legally be a management group rather than an individual, is responsible for the health and safety of the children in their care. The legal framework for registered early years settings is derived from both health and safety legislation and the national standards for under eights day care.

### Staff administering medicines

3 There is no legal or contractual duty on staff to administer medicine or supervise a child taking it. The only exceptions are set out in the paragraph below. Support staff may have specific duties to provide medical assistance as part of their contract. Of course, swift action needs to be taken by any member of staff to assist any child in an emergency. Employers should ensure that their insurance policies provide appropriate cover.

### Staff 'duty of care'

4 Anyone caring for children including teachers, other school staff and day care staff in charge of children have a common law duty of care to act like any reasonably prudent parent. Staff need to make sure

that children are healthy and safe. In exceptional circumstances the duty of care could extend to administering medicine and/or taking action in an emergency. This duty also extends to staff leading activities taking place off site, such as visits, outings or field trips.

## Admissions

5 Children with complex health needs have the same rights of admission to school as other children, and cannot generally be excluded from school for health reasons. In certain circumstances, eg where there is a risk to health and safety of staff or other pupils, children can be removed from school for health reasons. This, however, is not exclusion.

## The law

6 Legislation, notably the Education Act 1996, the Disability Discrimination Act 1995, the Care Standards Act 2000 and the Medicines Act 1968 are also relevant to schools and settings in dealing with children's complex health needs. The following paragraphs outline the provisions of these Acts that are relevant to the health and safety of children attending early years settings and schools.

## SEN and Disability Act (SENDA) 2001

7 The SEN and Disability Act (SENDA) 2001 amended Part IV of the Education Act 1996 making changes to the existing legislation, in particular strengthening the right of children with SEN to be educated in mainstream schools.

8 Schools and early years settings are both required to take 'reasonable steps' to meet the needs of disabled children.

## LEAs and Schools

9 SENDA also amended Part IV the Disability Discrimination Act (DDA) 1995 bringing access to education within the remit of the DDA, making it unlawful for schools and LEAs to discriminate against disabled pupils for a reason relating to their disability, without justification. This might include some children with complex health needs.

10 Part IV duties apply to all schools; private or state maintained, mainstream or special and those early years settings constituted as schools.

11 Some medical conditions may be classed as a disability. The responsible body of a school will need to consider what arrangements can reasonably be made to help support a pupil (or prospective pupil) who has a disability. The Disability Rights Commission has produced a Code of Practice for Schools. Advice

and training from local health professionals will help schools when looking at what arrangements they can reasonably make to support a pupil with a disability.

12 Since September 2002 schools and LEAs have been under a duty:
- not to treat less favourably disabled pupils or students, without justification, than pupils and students who are not disabled
- to make reasonable adjustments to ensure that disabled pupils and students are not put at a substantial disadvantage in comparison to those who are not disabled.

13 Schools are not, however, required to provide auxiliary aids or services or to make changes to physical features. Instead, schools and LEAs are under a duty to plan strategically to increase access, over time, to schools. This duty includes planning to increase access to the school premises, to the curriculum and providing written material in alternative formats to ensure accessibility.

14 Part IV duties cover discrimination in admissions, the provision of education and associated services and exclusions.

### Early years settings

15 Early years settings, not constituted as schools, must comply with Part 3 of the DDA; this includes day nurseries, family centres, pre-schools, playgroups and childminders (including those in a childminding network). The duties cover the refusal to provide a service, offering a lower standard of service or offering a service on worse terms to a disabled child.

16 Under Parts 3 and 4 of the DDA all settings are required not to treat a disabled child 'less favourably' than any other child for a reason relating to their disability. There may sometimes be justification for less favourable treatment, but it may not be possible to justify if there is a reasonable adjustment that might have been made but was not.

### Health and Safety at Work etc Act 1974

17 The Health and Safety at Work etc Act (HSWA) 1974 places duties on employers for the health and safety of their employees and anyone else on the premises. This covers the headteacher and teachers, non-teaching staff, children and visitors.[1]

18 Who the employer is depends on the type of school:
- for community schools, community special schools, voluntary controlled schools, maintained nursery schools and pupil referral units the employer is the local education authority (LEA)
- for foundation schools, foundation special schools and voluntary-aided schools the employer is the governing body
- for academies and city technology colleges the employer is the governing body

1 *Health and safety: responsibilities and powers* (DfES, 2001)

- for non-maintained special schools the employer is the trustees
- for other independent schools the employer is usually the governing body, proprietor or trustees

19 The employer for registered day care will depend on the way it has been set up. Settings may be run by private individuals, charities, voluntary committees, Local authorities, school governors, the proprietor or the trustees in some independent schools, and companies that provide day care as an additional service to customers (e.g. crèches in shops or sports clubs).

20 The employer of staff at a school or setting must do all that is reasonably practicable to ensure the health, safety and welfare of employees. The employer must also make sure that others, such as pupils and visitors, are not put at risk. The main actions employers must take under the Health and Safety at Work etc Act are to:
- prepare a written health and safety policy
- make sure that staff are aware of the policy and their responsibilities within that policy
- make arrangements to implement the policy
- make sure that appropriate safety measures are in place
- make sure that staff are properly trained and receive guidance on their responsibilities as employees

21 Most schools and settings will at some time have children on roll with complex health needs. The responsibility of the employer is to make sure that safety measures cover the needs of *all* children at the school or setting. This may mean making special arrangements for particular children.


### Management of Health and Safety at Work Regulations 1999

22 The Management of Health and Safety at Work Regulations 1999, made under the HSWA, require employers to:
- make an assessment of the risks of activities
- introduce measures to control these risks
- tell their employees about these measures

23 The national standards for day care settings make it clear that the registered person *must* comply with all relevant health and safety legislation. Registered persons in early years settings are also required under the national standards to take positive steps to promote safety. Supporting criteria under the safety standard includes undertaking risk assessments.

24 HWSA and the Management of Health and Safety at Work Regulations 1999 also apply to employees. Employees *must*:
- take reasonable care of their own and others health and safety
- co-operate with their employers
- carry out activities in accordance with training and instructions
- inform the employer of any serious risk

25 In some cases children with complex health needs may be more at risk than their classmates. Staff may need to take additional steps to safeguard the health and safety of such children. In a few cases individual procedures may be needed. The employer is responsible for making sure that all relevant staff know about and are, if necessary, trained to provide any additional support these children require.

### Manual Handling Operations Regulation 1992 (MHO)

26 The Manual Handling Operations Regulation 1992 were made under the Health and Safety at Work etc Act 1974 and to implement the European Directive 90/269/EEC (HSE 1992). They were part of a wider campaign to reduce back injuries. The regulations require employers to assess the risk in relation to manual handling, avoid manual handling operations which involve a risk of injury if possible, mechanise handling where that is possible and in all cases reduce risk to what is 'reasonably practicable'.

27 Reasonably practicable is defined as 'an employee has satisfied his/her duty if s/he can show that any further preventative steps would be grossly disproportionate to the further benefit that would accrue from their introduction (HSE 1992:8)'. The Regulation does not outlaw manual handling, it creates a hierarchy of measures for reducing the risks involved in manual handling.

28 Employers are required to:
- avoid manual handling operations which involve a risk of injury to employees
- assess remaining manual handling operations
- reduce the risk of injury
- provide general information on the weight of loads (this means children and young people)
- review the assessment

29 Employees are required to:
- make full and proper use of systems of work provided

30 Risk assessments for safer handling are clearly laid out in MHO 1992 known as the 'TILE' assessment and cover:
- the lifting task – why is it required, are there alternatives?
- the young person's weight and needs – it is *essential* to build in a section on how much the child or young person can do for themselves and how they could help in any handling activities.
- the physical environment, is it a safe place to lift, are there any hazards, is there sufficient space.
- the individual capacities of the lifter, is the carer/worker fit enough to lift, are they experienced, etc. This reinforces the need for health information on staff to ensure that they do not put themselves and the child at risk.

### Provision and Use of Work Equipment Regulations 1998 (PUWER)

31 There regulations apply to any equipment which is used by an employee at work, including equipment such as hoists, and set out employers' duty to ensure that equipment is:

- suitable for intended use
- safe for use
- used only by people who have received adequate information, instruction and training

### Lifting Operations and Lifting Equipment Regulations 1998 (LOLER)

32 These regulations contain specific requirements relating to equipment which is used by an employee at work which includes lifting equipment such as hoists and bath lifts. Employers have a duty to:

- provide training for staff on the use of all lifting equipment by a competent person
- provide instructions with the equipment
- ensure that equipment and accessories to lift people is checked by a competent person every six months
- carry out a risk assessment on the use of all equipment and make staff aware of the risks.

### Control of Substances Hazardous to Health Regulations 2002

33 The Control of Substances Hazardous to Health Regulations 2002 (COSHH) require employers to control exposures to hazardous substances to protect both employees and others. For example, Presept granules which are used for mopping up blood spillages.

### Misuse of Drugs Act 1971 and associated regulations

34 The supply, administration, possession and storage of certain drugs are controlled by the Misuse of Drugs Act 1971and associated regulations. This is of relevance to schools and settings because they may have a child that has been prescribed a controlled drug. The Regulations allow 'any person' to administer the drugs listed in the Regulations.

### Medicines Act 1968

35 The Medicines Act 1968 specifies the way that medicines are prescribed, supplied and administered within the UK and places restrictions on dealings with medicinal products, including their administration. Anyone may administer a prescribed medicine, with consent, to a third party, so long as it is in accordance with the prescriber's instructions. This indicates that a medicine may only be administered to the person for whom it has been prescribed,

labelled and supplied; and that no-one other than the prescriber may vary the dose and directions for administration.

36 The administration of prescription-only medicine by injection may be done by any person but must be in accordance with directions made available by a doctor, dentist, nurse prescriber or pharmacist prescriber in respect of a named patient.

### The Education (School Premises) Regulations 1999

37 The Education (School Premises) Regulations 1999 require every school to have a room appropriate and readily available for use for medical or dental examination and treatment and for the caring of sick or injured pupils. It *must* contain a washbasin and be reasonably near a water closet. It *must not* be teaching accommodation. If this room is used for other purposes as well as for medical accommodation, the body responsible *must* consider whether dual use is satisfactory or has unreasonable implications for its main purpose. The responsibility for providing these facilities in all maintained schools rests with the local authority.

38 The 1999 Regulations specify the accommodation provisions that apply to boarding schools only, these state that a boarding school must have one or more sick rooms.

### The Education (Independent Schools Standards) (England) Regulations 2003

39 The Education (Independent Schools Standards)(England) Regulations 2003 require that independent schools have and implement a satisfactory policy on First Aid and have appropriate facilities for pupils in accordance with the Education (School Premises) Regulations 1999.

### National standards for under eights day care and childminding – premises

40 The national standards do not require day care settings to have a separate first aid room but they do cover the promotion of good health and taking positive steps to prevent the spread of infection. Such settings should also have one washbasin for every ten children over two years of age.

41 The national standards also require premises to be safe, secure and suitable for their purpose. They must provide adequate space in an appropriate location, are welcoming to children and offer all the necessary facilities for a range of activities that promote their development. Supporting criteria under the standard includes space standards, outdoor play areas, toilets, staff facilities, kitchens and laundry facilities.

### Special Educational Needs – Education Act 1996

42 Section 312 of the Education Act 1996 sets out that a child has special educational needs if he has a learning difficulty that calls for special educational provision to be made for him. Children with complex health needs will not necessarily have special educational needs (SEN). For those who do, schools should refer to the DfES SEN guidance.[2]

43 Section 322 of the *Education Act 1996* requires that, upon request health authorities and primary care trusts *must* provide specific help to enable the LEA to exercise its statutory SEN functions unless the authority or trust consider that the specific help requested is not necessary to enable the LEA to exercise those functions or that it would not be reasonable to provide such help in the light of the resources available to them to exercise their statutory NHS functions. This applies whether or not a child attends a special school. Local authorities, schools and early years settings should work together, in close partnership with parents, to ensure proper support for children with complex health needs.

### Care Standards Act 2000

## Schools

44 Residential special schools are required to register with the Commission for Social Care Inspection (CSCI) and are subject to the requirements set out in the Children's Homes Regulations 2001. In respect of medicines, this is set out in Regulation 21 and places a duty on the registered person to make 'suitable arrangements for the recording, handling, safekeeping, safe administration and disposal of … medicines'. The Department of Health has also published National Minimum Standards (NMS) that set out guidance of how the Regulations may be met (Standard 13).

45 CSCI also works in conjunction with Ofsted to monitor health and social welfare in Boarding Schools. There are also NMS for Boarding Schools although such schools are not subject to Regulations under the Care Standards Act.

## Day care provision

46 The Children Act 1989 was amended by the Care Standards Act 2000 by the introduction of Part XA. In accordance with 79B in Part XA of the Children Act, the Office for Standards in Education (Ofsted) registers day care provision (day nurseries, crèches, out of school clubs and pre-school provision) and childminders. As regulator, Ofsted ensures that those who provide day care or childminding services are suitable and that the requirements set out in the national standards for under 8s day care and childminding are met. The registered person in early years settings

2 *SEN Code of Practice* (DfES, 2001) paragraphs 7:64–7:67.

in the private and voluntary sectors *must* meet the requirements of the national standards for under 8s day care and childminding.

47 The national standards for under 8s day care and childminding require that the registered person in an early years setting promotes the good health of children and takes positive steps to prevent the spread of infection and appropriate measures when they are ill (Standard 7).

48 The criteria for this standard sets out that the registered person has a clear policy, understood by all staff and discussed with parents, regarding the administration of medicines. If the administration of prescription medicine requires technical/medical knowledge then individual training *must* be provided for staff from a qualified health professional and that training *must* be specific to the individual child concerned.

49 There is a requirement in the national standards for under 8s day care and childminding that the registered person must take positive steps to promote safety within the setting and on outings and ensure proper precautions are taken to prevent accidents (Standard 6).

50 For day care settings, the criteria sets out that the registered person must take reasonable steps to ensure that hazards to children on the premises, both inside and outside, are minimised and is aware of, and complies with, health and safety regulations. Staff must be trained to have an understanding of health and safety requirements for the environment in which they work.

51 The national standards do not override the need for providers to comply with other legislation such as that covering health and safety, food hygiene and so on. The registered person would therefore need to be aware of all other legislative requirements as set out in this chapter.

# Appendix 3
# Research

### Prevalence of complex health needs

Although there are no national figures available on the prevalence of children with complex health needs there is a consensus amongst paediatricians, social services managers and educationalists that the population of children using services now is radically different from ten years ago (Russell et al, 2002).

There have been a number of studies in the area of children who are dependent of technology. In a report commissioned by the Department of Health, Glendinning estimated that there were 6,000 technology dependent children living in the United Kingdom (Glendinning *et al,* 1999). This figure is now likely to be significantly higher. There is limited information about prevalence and trends relating to specific procedures within this group. A study by Townsley and Robinson (2000) estimated that the number of children under the age of 15 years fed via a tube rose by nearly 60%, from 519 to 887 between 1994 and 1996. In 1977, 136 children under the age of 16 years were registered as needing long-term ventilation. This figure rose to 241 children in 2000, as increase of 77% in three years. (Ludvigsen and Morrison, 2003).

Three research studies in recent years which inform our understanding and knowledge of this area are:
* Study conducted in 2004 by Tricia Nash at Exeter University on the provision of medical and nursing support in schools and colleges in the South West of England for children with life-limiting or life-threatening conditions.
* Research work conducted by the Social Policy Research Unit at York University. The initial study investigated the need for support in schools in order to meet the needs of children with health needs (Lightfoot *et al,* 1998). A follow up study focused on improving communication between health providers and schools (Mukherjee *et al,* 2000).
* Research study, *Meeting medical needs in mainstream education*, carried out by the National Children's Bureau (Data, J. and Ryder, N. 2005). This research project looked at how mainstream secondary schools meet the needs of students who have a medical condition. The study focused on 17 schools based in two local authorities and included a survey of over 6500 students as well as detailed case studies.

Further details are contained in the References section of this handbook.

# References

Datta, J and Ryder, N. 2005. *Meeting medical needs in mainstream education*. London: NCB.

Department for Education and Skills. 2001. *Special educational needs. Code of practice*. London: DfES.

Department for Education and Skills and Department of Health. 2004. *National service framework for children, young people and maternity services. Medicines for children and young people*. London: DoH.

Department for Education and Skills and Department of Health. 2005. *Managing medicines in schools and early years settings*. London: DfES.

Department of Health. 2000. *Good practice in continence services*.

Glendinning, C, Kirk, S, Guiffrida, A and Lawton, D. 1999. *The community-based care of technology dependent children in the UK: definitions, numbers and costs*. Research Report commissioned by the Social Care Group, Department of Health. Manchester: National Primary Care Research and Development Centre.

Health and Safety Executive 1992. *Manual Handling Operations Regulations (MHOR)*. HMSO

Lenehan, C., Morrison, J. and Stanley, J. 2004. *The dignity of risk. A practical handbook for professionals working with disabled children and their families*. London: Council for Disabled Children.

Lightfoot, J., Wright, S. and Sloper, P. (1998). *Service support for children with a chronic illness or physical disability attending mainstream schools*. NHS1576. York: Social Policy Research Unit. University of York.

Ludvigsen, A. and Morrison, J. May 2003. *Breathing space. Community support for children on long-term ventilation*. Essex: Barnardos.

Mukherjee, S., Lightfoot, J. and Sloper, P. 2000. *Improving communication between health and education for children with chronic illnesses or physical disability*. NHS1740. York: Social Policy Research Unit. University of York.

Nash, T. and Asprey, A. October 2004. *Children with life-limiting or life-threatening illnesses and their support in schools and colleges: the provision of medical and nursing support. Part 1. Parent interviews*. Exeter: Department of Sociology. University of Exeter.

Russell, P., Lenehan, C., Castle, K,. Dawkins, B. and Smith, P. October 2002. *The policies and Practice of resucitation: an in-depth study of the lessons to be learned from events at Ysgol Crug Glas: Report to the National Assembly for Wales.* London: Council for Disabled Children.

Townsley, R. and Robinson, C. 2001. *Food for thought?* Bristol: Norah Fry Research Centre, University of Bristol.

# Resources

### Communication passports

Millar, S. and Aitken, S. 2003. *Personal Communication Passports: Guidelines for good practice.* Edinburgh: CALL Centre.

Nottinghamshire Inclusion Project. *Passports – Frameworks for sharing information about a child with others.* Nottinghamshire LEA SEN Inclusion Team.

### Continence

See web for guidance on continence: www.dh.gov.uk/PublicationsAndStatistics/Publications/Publications PolicyAndGuidance/PublicationsPolicyAndGuidanceArticle/fs/en? CONTENT_ID=4005851&chk=ozVeMn

*Leicester City's continence policy* – a good example that can be adapted for local use: http://www.surestart.gov.uk/publications/

*Managing a child with bladder and bowel problems in school – A resource pack* This includes basic information on the common toileting and bowel and bladder problems including definitions, prevalence and how it would affect the child in school in terms of management. The pack contains suggested templates for the development of training packages for staff to enable them to meet the individual needs of children requiring help and support in school. Available from www.promocon.co.uk

### Disability Discrimination Act

Stobbs, P. and Rieser, R. 2002. *Making it work. Removing disability discrimination. Are you ready?* London: National Children's Bureau.

*Early years and the Disability Discrimination Act 1995 – what service providers need to know* can be downloaded from www.surestart.gov.uk/publications/

### First aid

*Guidance on First Aid in Schools.* www.teachernet.gov.uk/firstaid.

## General information on health conditions

### Contact a Family

209–211 City Road, London EC1V 1JN

*tel* 020 7608 8700    *fax* 020 7608 8701

*e-mail* info@cafamily.org.uk    www.cafamily.org.uk

**Early Support Programme**  This programme was set up to improve services to babies and very young disabled children and their families. It has developed a range of materials for pre-school children. Details can be found at www.earlysupport.org.uk

## Life-threatening and life-limiting conditions

ACT. 2004. *Integrated multi-agency care pathways for children with life-threatening and life-limiting conditions.* Bristol: ACT. (www.act.org.uk)

## Long-term ventilation

Noyes, J. and Lewis, M. 2005. *From hospital to home. Guidance on discharge management and community support for children using long-term ventilation.* London: Barnardos.

## Residential schools

Children's Residential Network. 2004. *Towards shared good practice – Providers and regulators together: A development pack to support providers meet the requirements of Standard 13 – 'Treatment and administration of medicines within the home'.* www.ncb.org.uk/networks/crn then click on 'Document library'

Morgan, R. 2004. *Young person's guide to the Residential Special Schools Standards.* London: National Children's Bureau and DfES.

Stanley, J. 2004. *Parent's guide to the Residential Special Schools Standards.* London: National Children's Bureau and DfES.

Williams, A. 2004. *Staff guide to the Residential Special Schools Standards.* London: National Children's Bureau and DfES.

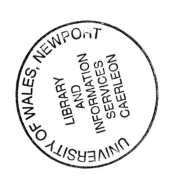